Dyslexia or
Illiteracy?

Open University Press
Children With Special Needs Series

Editors

PHILLIP WILLIAMS
Emeritus Professor of Education,
University College of North Wales, Bangor.

PETER YOUNG
Formerly Tutor in the education of children with
learning difficulties, Cambridge Institute of Education;
educational writer, researcher and consultant.

This is a series of short and authoritative introductions for parents, teachers, professionals and anyone concerned with children with special needs. The series will cover the range of physical, sensory, mental, emotional and behavioural difficulties, and the changing needs from infancy to adult life in the family, at school and in society. The authors have been selected for their wide experience and close professional involvement in their particular fields. All have written penetrating and practical books readily accessible to non-specialists.

TITLES IN THE SERIES

Dyslexia or Illiteracy?

Realizing the right to read

Peter Young and Colin Tyre

Open University Press
Milton Keynes · Philadelphia

Open University Press
Celtic Court
22 Ballmoor
Buckingham
MK18 1XW.

and

1900 Frost Road, Suite 101
Bristol, PA 19007, USA

First published 1983
Reprinted 1986, 1987, 1990

Copyright © 1983 Open University Press

British Library Cataloguing in Publication Data

Young, Peter
    Dyslexia or Illiteracy?—(Children with special
    needs series)
    1. Dyslexia   2. Reading disability
    I. Title   II. Tyre, Colin   III. Series
    371.9'14   LB1050.5

    ISBN 0-335-10192-5
    ISBN 0-335-10191-7 Pbk

Printed in Great Britain by St Edmundsbury Press Limited
Bury St Edmunds, Suffolk

Contents

Editor's Introduction

Education depends heavily on the ability to read. Most of us gain and extend this deceptively simple skill during our first few years at school, but for a minority of children reading is a skill which is never or perhaps only partially acquired. The difficulties experienced by this minority cause understandable concern to parents and to teachers and largely account for the long history of research into the learning and teaching of reading.

But the history of reading research is not only long — it is also controversial. All work with children with special needs requires collaboration between specialists, and usually collaboration is smooth and untroubled. But, in this case, the problem of understanding and dealing with children's reading difficulties, there has been a long-standing difference between the followers of two alternative approaches. One is in origin a medically-based approach believing in the existence of a "condition" called dyslexia, whereas the other is in origin an educational/psychological approach, believing that reading difficulty is one example of the many kinds of learning difficulties children show. The debate between these two schools of thought has been both lengthy and at times fierce and it is with this debate and its consequences for helping children with reading problems that this book is concerned.

Peter Young and Colin Tyre review this topic from a post-Warnock Report position. They believe that ". . . of paramount importance are the needs of the children, not the labels attached to them". From this standpoint they make a strong plea for forgetting apparent differences and uniting to attack the real difficulties of reading.

The book broaches this theme in a short introductory chapter and then moves on to discuss the various usages and meanings of the term dyslexia and the numbers of children involved. Chapter 3 offers a particularly vivid description of the process of learning to read, firmly rooted in the acquisition of language in all its aspects, and linked especially with speech and writing. The authors present their own "holistic" view of the reading process as a helpful model.

The next two chapters cover and comment on a selection of research questions and the book ends with two chapters which indicate some approaches to the diagnosis and treatment of reading difficulties. The material is illustrated by the results of the authors' own action research designed to help children, including those diagnosed by independent specialists as dyslexic, with serious reading problems. Of particular interest is the emphasis placed on enlisting and harnessing the support and energies of the parents, on the importance of parents and teachers working in harmony, and the resulting changes in children's performance and motivation.

At a time when standards of reading and literacy are once more in the forefront of national debate, the problems of children who are retarded in reading are again matters of national concern. Peter Young and Colin Tyre offer a way forward from the arid sterility of the dyslexia/reading difficulty controversy. They offer a new look at an old problem. And they write in clear and fluent prose which will engage the interest of both parent and professional.

Phillip Williams

CHAPTER 1

What Seems to be the Problem?

"What seems to be the problem?"
"It's these squiggly black marks — they
don't make any sense to me!"

Making sense of print is the only problem some children are said to have. They find everything else straightforward but, for some obscure reason, find learning to read and spell virtually impossible. Their problem, a comparatively minor and rare one in the spectrum of mental, sensory and physical defects, disabilities and handicaps, has been variously labelled. Terms such as word-blindness, strephosymbolia (twisted symbols), specific developmental or congenital dyslexia and specific reading retardation syndrome are handled about as if everyone knew what they really meant. The handicapped, like the poor — or socially disadvantaged, economically deprived or underdeveloped — may have little done to help them but they do attract splendid vocabularies. These children with reading problems have also attracted extensive research, a considerable literature, public interest, heated controversy and litigation. One reason for this, of course, is the importance of reading in our culture. Another reason is the interest of the medical, psychological and educational professions in the nature, causes and treatment of the problem. Particularly significant has been the active concern of the parents of these children.

Many parents complain that they have been misunderstood, treated cavalierly and labelled as over-anxious trouble-makers when they have sought help for their children. Often they have

1

been dismayed at the lack of facilities and the ineffectiveness of what help has been given. As one father complained, "They can put men on the moon and teach chimpanzees sign-language — but they can't teach my son to read!" Examining the difficulties experienced by the parents illuminates many of the difficulties and needs of the children. It also highlights the problem of understanding what is meant by dyslexia.

Parents expect their children to learn to read. The parents of these children are understandably dismayed that they can't.

The Milestones of Reading

Throughout a child's life parents recognize achievements or milestones which have a particular significance. "Joan cut her first tooth!" "John pulled himself up!" "Jill can walk!" "Jack said his first word!" Milestones such as these are important in themselves. They signal that the child is growing and developing normally. They reassure parents, too, that there is harmony between the child's needs and the conditions and nurture they are providing. As each milestone is passed, at more or less the right time and in more or less the right order, parents' hopes for their children's future growth and development are confirmed and strengthened. The first word will lead to sentences and to conversation. And, somewhere along that line of development, will come the milestone of reading.

Of all the milestones, reading is the most difficult to place chronologically. Children usually start reading somewhere between the ages of three and eight years. Whenever we place it, there will be some perfectly normal people who began reading earlier or later than those rough limits. This brings us to the first problem encountered by parents of children with reading difficulties. At what age is it reasonable to become concerned if a child is not reading?

Whenever a child starts reading, it is seen as a particularly important milestone. Like the ability to use spoken language, learning to read demonstrates the development of intellect, the ability to learn, the mastery of complex skills and the child's growing self-reliance and independence. Reading gives the child access to education, to the world of books and information and to our culture. The child is out of the trap of illiteracy. More immediately, reading will contribute to the development of language and, through the related skills of handwriting and spelling, to communication and expression in written language. For the child it often seems like magic. For parents it is confirmation that they have provided the right encouragement, the right informal and formal education for their children, and that their children are competent and intelligent pupils who will be able to take full advantage of their schooling.

When a child whose development has hitherto been normal fails to learn to read, the parents' realization that something is wrong only comes gradually. This is not only because of the broad age-span in which a child may learn to read but also because learning to read involves the gradual bringing together of a variety of skills. The child has had to learn the shapes and sounds of letters, to attack reading from left to right and to build up sounds and words to make sense. So parents encourage, wait for all the pieces of the jigsaw to drop into place — and hope. Often they have to go on hoping for a long time, hoping that all will be well once the child starts school, changes class, gets a new teacher, changes method or moves up to the next school. When, at last, they realize that their children appear to be struggling against insuperable odds, they are perplexed and alarmed. They fear for their children's future, worry about how they will cope with examinations, see them falling further and further behind, and are filled with doubt and uncertainty. Haven't they talked enough, read to their children enough, stimulated and encouraged enough? Or have they done too much? Are their children less able than they thought, their swans ducks? Have they missed some vital clue? Is sight or hearing defective? Is the child lazy and inattentive at school? Is it heredity — a family failing?

Past, present and future are all put in doubt when a child fails to learn to read. For the parents, rightly and inevitably, the problem is charged with anxiety and emotion. They would be remarkably unfeeling and uncaring parents were this not the case. Yet some parents have been told that their anxieties are the cause of their children's problems. Frequently, when they have turned to schools for help, they have been told to be patient, to wait and not to worry. But this advice they often found unacceptable because it denied their own intimate perceptions of their children and their difficulties. Often parents have had their children's sight and hearing tested, sought the advice of doctors and of educational or clinical psychologists, agreed that their children receive remedial help, all without any significant new factor being discovered or any appreciable improvement being made in the children's reading.

A Case of Categorization

It is often during this process, when they are most anxious and vulnerable, that parents become aware of terms like specific developmental dyslexia and specific reading retardation syndrome, which suggest a new world of scientific knowledge, specialist skills and new hope. Unfortunately, it soon becomes apparent that these words appear to mean different things to different people. The experts do not agree amongst themselves and the esoteric skills look like print prodding and phonics. Worse, the words are categories, labels, seemingly vested with legal significance, and on them depend the kinds of help the children may or may not be given. Accept one label and the local education authority will provide help. Accept another label and the parents may have to pay for tuition themselves and travel long distances to get it.

Whatever the outcome, one thing is usually confirmed: the children need help. For some that specialist help, whether from the local education authority remedial centre or from a specialist clinic, produces results. For some it is a question of too little help too late. For others, comes the realization that the children will need help and understanding all their lives.

The history of the struggles and successes of parents to get help and understanding for these children is well-documented. Like the parents of cerebral palsied, autistic, mentally handicapped, spina bifida and other handicapped children, they found that the only way they could get help was by forming voluntary associations, arousing public concern and convincing central and local government that their children had a distinct category of handicap which justified distinctive specialist educational treatment. The parents of these children with reading difficulties could not have undertaken their difficult task at a less propitious time. They have campaigned to get dyslexia recognized as a category of handicap at the very time when many parents of handicapped children in North America and some in the UK were campaigning, together with other interested people, to get categories of handicap abolished and to get children out of special schools and classes and into ordinary schools and the mainstream of education.

Yet, so successful were the parents and their associations in England and Wales that the Chronically Sick and Disabled Persons Act, 1970, a private member's measure, gave brief parliamentary recognition to the term "dyslexia". In sections 25–27, it required local education authorities, so far as was practicable, to provide for, amongst others, "acutely dyslexic children", in maintained or assisted schools. However, this modification of the 1944 Education Act was overtaken by the Education Act of 1976, then by the Government White Paper, "Special Needs in Education", 1980, and the Education Act, 1981. Categories were dropped, labelling of children was no longer a prerequisite for special education.

Special Educational Needs — Not Categories

In place of categories, legislation in England and Wales has endorsed the recommendation of the Warnock Committee's Report, *Special Educational Needs*, for a wider concept of handicap "which focuses on the special educational needs of a child rather than on the possible physical, mental or emotional causes of the handicap". The distinction between special and remedial education and the question of categories are no longer central issues. What are of paramount importance are the needs of the children, not the labels attached to them. However, so far as children with severe difficulties in learning to read were concerned, the Warnock Report made specific recommendations. While recognizing the need for "programmes to meet the requirements of this group of children", about whom it had "received much evidence from dyslexia associations", the Report made it clear that, rather than call them dyslexic, it preferred to designate them as children having "specific learning difficulties in reading, writing and spelling".

Many of the parents of these children, the voluntary dyslexia associations and some of the specialists involved with the diagnosis and treatment of the problem, are dissatisfied with this desig-nation. They point out that whereas handicaps such as blindness, deafness and mental defects are accepted, there is still argument about dyslexia as a handicap. Voluntary associations have redoubled their efforts to establish centres for dyslexic pupils. Many parents believe that, because the term dyslexia is not accepted, the needs of their children will not be fully met. They are alarmed that the Department of Education and Science, local education authorities, the ombudsmen, many educational psychologists and members of the medical profession reject the use of the term dyslexia in favour of "specific learning difficulties in reading, writing and spelling".

It is claimed that these children's difficulties are different from those of children who are retarded in reading by lack of general ability or "intelligence". They are also held to be different from those whose difficulties are the result of social and linguistic deprivation or of emotional and behavioural problems. But, like these children, they nonetheless have reading problems. It is said that dyslexic children nevertheless differ since their difficulties are constitutional and intractable, and are exclusively or largely limited to reading and its associated skills.

Many people find this a difficult concept to accept. They point to the fact that an enormous variety of factors can cause difficulties in reading and suggest that these may well account for the problems these children have. Moreover, they point to the fact that many of the constitutional factors which have been brought forward to account for the difficulties of these children, exist in children who are successful readers.

It is the purpose of this book to look at the theories of dyslexia, at the research and the arguments, and to attempt to contribute to the understanding of these children. However, we will do so in the context of a much wider concern for the literacy of all children. The basis of the concept of special educational needs is that "education is a good, and a specifically human good, to which all human beings are entitled". Literacy, the foundation of our educational system, is a specifically human good to which all are entitled as of right. In examining dyslexia in children, at a time when the categorization of handicaps is no longer the determining factor in whether or not pupils' special needs should be met, it is timely to look at the problem objectively, to put it in this broader perspective of the needs of all children for literacy, and to look in some detail at the reading process itself.

However, what seems to be very much the matter is that "dyslexia" has caused as much confusion among those who have espoused or eschewed its use as reading has caused the children.

CHAPTER 2

The Problem of the Difficulty

**"We shouted and screamed at each other, noted new and
surprising similarities between our patients . . ."
Max Coltheart, Karalyn Patterson and John C. Marshall,
Preface to _Deep Dyslexia_ (1980)**

Just as dyspepsia has been called "the remorse of a guilty
stomach", so dyslexia has been called "middle-class illiteracy". The
words and their uses have a lot in common. _Dys-_ means _having
difficulty with_, and dyspepsia means _having difficulty with digest-
ion_. Dyslexia means _having difficulty with reading and spelling
language_. The words mean more or less what they say — in Greek.
However, not everyone agrees that this dictionary meaning is
correct so far as dyslexia is concerned and, because it is of such
recent usage, the word is only beginning to get established in
dictionaries and has had some unfortunate definitions in some of
them. The arguments about the meaning of the word revolve
around the wisdom or otherwise of defining it as _having difficulty
with language_. While we fully agree that dyslexia is clearly a disorder involving language no useful purpose is served in defining it
so vaguely. The word is vague enough as it is. For if we tell a doctor
that we have dyspepsia or dyslexia in both instances he will still
want to know, "What seems to be the matter?" Neither word is
precise or specific. The conditions can be very mild or very severe
and anywhere in between. And, just as dyspepsia has a variety of
causes from cucumber to ulcers, so dyslexia may have a variety of
causes.

Acquired Dyslexia

Dyslexia is a made up, work-horse of a term used originally by the medical profession to describe the reading and spelling difficulties of patients who had suffered certain sorts of brain damage. The brain damage may have been caused in accidents or wars or as the result of tumours, strokes, psychiatric disorders, drugs or the effects of ageing. It is synonymous with the term "word-blindness" which was introduced at the end of the nineteenth century and was particularly appropriate later when used by ophthalmologists and others who believed that reading difficulties were caused by some form of visual defect or by the way in which the brain processed visual images. Today, the term dyslexia properly belongs to such members of the medical profession as neurologists, psychiatrists and to clinical psychologists and neuropsychologists working with them. Dyslexia is not a disease, but a term used to describe the symptoms of damage to the brain: the impairment of the function of reading. Some patients will have difficulties only in reading and spelling long and unusual words; some will be unable to recognize the letters of the alphabet. Some patients will have difficulty with the "little words" of langauge such as "to, is, by, but". Some will have difficulty in reading aloud; others will read aloud but fail to understand what they have read. Increasingly, specialists distinguish not merely between degrees of difficulty in reading or spelling or writing but also between kinds of dyslexia such as deep, surface, central, semantic, auditory and visual. In all the cases of *acquired* dyslexia the specialists can point to hard signs or to soft signs to support the view that the difficulties are in some way caused by brain damage. *Hard* signs are, for instance, the physical injury or wound to the brain itself, the evidence revealed by an operation or autopsy or other evidence which may show that there have been cerebral lesions or haemorrhage as in a stroke. *Soft* signs are provided by unusual EEG (electroencephalogram) patterns, abnormal reflexes or difficulties with hand-eye co-ordination and orientation, for example.

Developmental Dyslexia

When medical specialists began studying reading, spelling and writing difficulties in otherwise healthy and normal children they had to distinguish between these children and the cases of acquired dyslexia. This they did by describing the children as cases of *specific developmental dyslexia* or *congenital dyslexia*. These rather ambiguous terms are used to indicate that the children's difficulties are constitutional and not the result of some primary handicap of the mind or of the senses, or of lack of educational opportunity. Specific developmental dyslexia is intended to suggest, not that the dyslexia has developed, but that there may have been a developmental lag, some failure of neural maturation, which accounts for the children's difficulties. Congenital dyslexia simply means that the child appears to have been born with the difficulties. Of course, many handicapped children have dyslexic problems which can be directly attributed to their primary handicaps, such as cerebral palsy and spina bifida, but the numbers of these handicapped children who are also dyslexic are much smaller than one might expect, having regard to the severity of the physical dysfunctions with which they are afflicted. For the moment, however, we wish to focus attention on those children who are said to have specific developmental or congenital dyslexia and no other defects directly or indirectly associated with their reading, spelling and writing difficulties.

Unlike cases of acquired dyslexia, specific developmental dyslexia is not supported by hard or soft signs of brain damage in the majority of cases. It is also different from acquired dyslexia in another very important respect: acquired dyslexia means that the patient is no longer able to perform skills in which he or she was previously proficient, whereas a child said to be a case of specific developmental dyslexia has difficulty *in learning* the skill. Although a child may have no difficulty in learning other skills, and cannot be said to have a general learning difficulty, it is not unreasonable to suppose that a child may have a specific learning difficulty so far as reading or writing or spelling are concerned. Some of us have difficulties in learning to play a musical instrument or to swim. We accept that, in the spectrum of human diversity, some people have perfect pitch and others are tone deaf, some are colour-blind and others are allergic. Maureen C. aged 6 years was rescued from a fate worse than dyslexia when she was found to be allergic to the glue used in the binding of a certain series of reading books. Unless careful thought and investigation is given to the possibility that the difficulties may lie in the learning of the task or in some component of the task itself — whether it be an antipathy to the methods, books or materials being used, or to the teacher — we are failing to recognize the complexity of children's needs. We shall have to return to this problem later for, as we have already observed, reading involves the bringing together and mastery of a number of skills. Moreover, it could be argued, that if a child responds fairly readily to changes of method and materials and learns to read, it is extremely unlikely that there pre-existed any dyslexic constitutional condition in any meaningful medical sense. However, children with intractable reading difficulties do exist, and some of them have spelling difficulties which may be more difficult to deal with than their reading problems. In this connection it should be remembered that the majority of proficient readers can read and understand more words than they can spell correctly. We should not be surprised at beginning readers who are having difficulty in learning to read who also have even greater difficulty in spelling. Do we need a medical explanation and a medical term for their difficulties?

Within a medical context the use of the terms "dyslexia" or "acquired dyslexia" presents no problem. As terms which are understood by specialists working in similar or related fields they can be understood and the conditions can be described in as much detail as the circumstances demand. The further the terms are removed from a medical context the less they mean. Much of the controversy and confusion over the use of the word dyslexia when applied to children's difficulties has arisen because people expect it to be precise, specific and scientific, which it certainly is not. It is nothing but a word to describe difficulties over a wide range of skills involved in reading. It cannot be defined more accurately than that. But, of course, when a medical term is used to describe children's difficulties we cannot be blamed for assuming that it is used with medical justification. It is also reasonable to expect an adequate description of its causes and effects.

Circular Definitions

At first sight, the description of specific developmental dyslexia by the World Federation of Neurology, 1968, appears unexceptional:

a disorder in children who, despite conventional classroom experience, fail to attain the language skills of reading, writing and
spelling commensurate with their intellectual abilities.

In fact, this description is circular: children with difficulties in
reading and spelling etc. "fail to attain" reading and spelling skills.
The description rightly makes the point that the skills are language
skills and not just mechanical skills but it tells us nothing about the
degree or extent, cause or effect of the difficulties. Significantly, the
difficulties have become a disorder, however.

In the description used by the British Dyslexia Association the
difficulties have become a disability:

A dyslexic person is one who has a specific language disability
affecting spelling, reading and other language skills characterised
by a discrepancy between his mental potential and his educational
level despite conventional classroom instruction and despite
absence of any primary emotional trouble or adverse environmental
condition.

Again we have a circular argument and what amounts to little more
than a description of someone who is underachieving in reading.
How severe are these "disabilities" and how great are the "dis-
crepancies"? The only meaningful way in which dyslexia can be
described is by stating precisely what the specific reading, writing
and spelling difficulties are in each case, and by delineating exactly
what the individual child can and cannot do. Certainly specialists
who have associated themselves with general descriptions such as
these have served a useful purpose in alerting us to the fact that
some children may have constitutional difficulties preventing them
from making progress. In that respect they are making political
rather than medical statements.

Different Perspectives

Another reason for confusion over the use of the term "dyslexia" is
the difference in background and experience between the medical
and the educational professions. A doctor who examines a child
with reading difficulties will notice the similarities between the
child's problems and those of his patients with acquired dyslexia.

An educational psychologist examining the same child will notice the similarities between the child's problems and those of hundreds of other children he has taught and examined. However, the doctor may well be able to build up a picture of a number of other "soft" signs which suggest the child is dyslexic. The child may confuse left and right, write clumsily and not be able to repeat a series of five digits in reverse order. Here the doctor is recognizing a significant cluster of symptoms, a syndrome, which has been noted in other patients. The educational psychologist, noting these difficulties, would attach less importance to them because his training and experience indicate that they are difficulties experienced by many children who are proficient readers. The doctor is perfectly justified in saying the child has dyslexic problems, if he means simply that the child has reading, spelling and writing difficulties. The educational psychologist is equally justified in remarking that, for an 8-year-old, the child is of average ability in reading and spelling. This problem of the different perspectives is nicely brought out by one of the contributors to the book quoted at the head of this chapter. Writing about "surface dyslexic" patients who have difficulty with the spelling-to-sound characteristics of words, Tony Marcel writes:

> Something which, surprisingly, nobody seems to have commented on is the striking similarity between the attempts to read single words by surface dyslexic patients and the attempts made by beginning readers. Two phenomena spring to mind quite readily. One is that children will often guess words with two constraints — that most of the letters should be accounted for phonetically and that the guess is probably in the child's spoken vocabulary. . . . The second phenomenon is related to this and is that the child laboriously attempts to sound out the elements of the word in order, often making several attempts.

It is indeed surprising that so little research has been directed to examining the similarities between the strategies used by beginning readers and those used by dyslexic patients. As Marcel later observes of a study of some cases of developmental dyslexia in four boys aged 9 to 13: "Is it possible that the boys classified as dyslexic . . . had merely not yet learnt the appropriate specifications (for sounding certain words) rather than had a disability? . . . If the problems of "development dyslexics" of this type are not insuperable, then maybe those of traumatic dyslexics of this type are not either."

It is our view that there is everything to be gained by in-depth research which is informed by experience drawn from both normal and abnormal learning and performance. However, there are dangers in jumping from the clinic to the classroom without making some reservations and provisos.

How to be dyslexic without difficulty

A few years ago The Dyslexia Institute in England published a pamphlet entitled "Recognising the Dyslexic Child". The reader was told that if the answer to three or four of the following questions is "yes", it is quite possible that the "child is appreciably handicapped by dyslexia".

If he is aged 12 or over
Are there still occasional inaccuracies in reading?
Is his spelling still somewhat odd looking?
Do instructions, telephone numbers, etc. sometimes have to be repeated?
Does he get "tied up" in saying long words? (Try him with *preliminary, philosophical, statistical.*)
Is he sometimes confused over times and dates?
Is a lot of checking needed before he can copy things accurately?
Does he still have difficulty with the harder arithmetic tables?
In reciting arithmetic tables in the traditional way . . . does he "lose his place", "skip" some of the numbers, or forget what point he has reached?
Present him with four digits, e.g. 4-9-5-8, spoken at one second intervals, to say in reverse order.
Does he slip back to some of his earlier habits when he is tired?

It is doubtful if many escaped that net! Strangely, for a questionnaire about reading and spelling difficulties, only the first two questions refer to them and much of it reads more like a means of identifying cases of dyscalculia — difficulties with arithmetic.

In fact, all the factors mentioned in the questionnaire have been identified by Professor Miles, in his book *Understanding Dyslexia*, as significant in children who are experiencing reading and spelling difficulties. This may well be so, but, if it is, one is scarcely justified in taking the factors out of context and claiming that combined with "occasional inaccuracies in reading" they constitute a *handicap*. It is not surprising that the dyslexia lobby has attracted such support and found so much concern among parents when children could be so readily labelled both "dyslexic" and "handicapped".

Specific Difficulties

In England and Wales, in response to the twin pressures from parents in the dyslexia associations and from the local education authorities anxious to have the position clarified, the Department of Education and Science instructed the Advisory Committee on Handicapped Children to investigate developmental dyslexia. This Report (1972) concluded that there were no agreed criteria for distinguishing children said to be dyslexic from other pupils with reading difficulties. It agreed that there were many reasons for perceptual and learning difficulties in reading and that there were children whose reading difficulties could not be accounted for by lack of ability, lack of schooling or by emotional troubles. It failed to find one group of symptoms or characteristics which could be singled out, but recognized that there were a number of different patterns of difficulties among pupils who found problems in learning to read and spell. The Report recommended that these pupils with severe and long-term reading and spelling difficulties should be described as *"children with specific reading difficulties"*.

The views and recommendations of that Report were endorsed by the Bullock Committee of Inquiry into the teaching of English, *A Language for Life*, 1975. It recommended that, "the great majority of children with reading difficulties should be given the help they need in their own schools", but those children who experienced severe difficulties in learning to read "often referred to as 'dyslexic'" were likely to need more intensive treatment which might best be given in "a remedial centre or reading clinic, a facility which should be available in every authority. They should be able to offer, or at least have access to, a comprehensive diagnostic service, calling as necessary upon the skills of doctor and psychologist to complement the skills of an experienced staff of teachers."

The Bullock Report also considered the term dyslexic "not

susceptible to precise operational definition" and for this reason and, as it did not "indicate any clearly defined course of treatment", proposed a more helpful term *"specific reading retardation"*. This is defined as:

> A syndrome characterised by severe reading difficulties which are not accountable for in terms of low intelligence and which are not explicable merely in terms of the lower end of a normal distribution of reading skills.

Here the term *retardation* is used to describe under-achievement in reading after both the age and the intelligence of the child are taken into account. Rutter and Yule, who developed this definition and the statistical methods by which pupils may be tested and identified, had found that 4% of the 10-year-old age group in the classic study of children on the Isle of Wight exhibited this syndrome and were 28 months or more retarded in reading. In an inner London borough, 10% of the 10-year-olds were similarly retarded. The children were not a homogeneous group and in some cases it was not possible to determine precisely either the cause or the nature of their basic disability. Rutter and Yule considered these pupils to be both quantitatively and qualitatively different from the kinds of pupils one would expect to find at the lower ability levels in reading. Boys were over three times as commonly affected as girls and pupils often had speech, language and spelling difficulties. Many had problems of verbal coding, such as remembering the names of the months in order. Follow-up studies showed that, unless the children were given special help, they were unlikely to have improved by the time they were due to leave school.

The reader will have noticed that the description of the syndrome is similar in a number of respects to the characteristics of developmental dyslexia. Rutter and Yule's work is valuable to schools, local education authorities and researchers in that they explain their criteria in detail, together with the tests and the statistical procedures they use, so that, whether one agrees with them or not, at least one knows the basis on which their conclusions are founded. Moreover, they have shown that these children who are severely retarded in reading exist in all social classes and at all levels of ability. Using their, or similar, methods it is possible for schools and LEAs to identify these pupils and plan the teachers, resources and medical and psychological expertise to identify and to meet individual needs.

In the past, because of their concern for the classification of dyslexia as a category of handicap, the dyslexia associations, and many of the specialists associated with them, rejected both the terms "specific reading difficulties" and "specific reading retardation syndrome". It was to be hoped that in future they would have less objection to one or other of these terms which mean precisely the same as dyslexia in English! There is no doubt that some children have intractable difficulties in learning to read and spell and in other aspects of language. Whether one calls them dyslexic or not doesn't matter, so long as we accept that the children have reading difficulties.

The Indefinable

However, with the appearance of the terms "learning difficulty" and "disability" in the Warnock Report in which there is a recommendation for a more discriminating approach to the needs of these children, Dr MacDonald Critchley, the clinical neurologist whose work on behalf of dyslexic children for a number of decades has given him an international reputation, has made a valiant attempt to define what many say is "the indefinable":

> Developmental dyslexia is a learning disability which initially shows itself by difficulty in learning to read, and later by erratic spelling and by lack of facility in manipulating written as opposed to spoken words. The condition is cognitive in essence, and usually genetically determined. It is not due to intellectual inadequacy or to lack of socio-cultural opportunity, or to emotional factors, or to any known structural brain-defect. It probably represents a specific maturational defect which tends to lessen as the child grows older, and is capable of considerable improvement, especially when appropriate remedial help is afforded at the earliest opportunity.

This definition attempts to establish developmental dyslexia as a condition which is cognitive in essence and which "probably represents a maturational lag". Certainly, it argues the case for these children to be considered as falling within the provisions of the Education Act 1981 which states that a child has a learning difficulty if he has a significantly greater difficulty in learning than the majority of children or has a disability which either prevents or hinders him from making use of educational facilities of a kind generally provided in schools. With this we doubt if many would quarrel: if children have severe difficulties in learning to read then there is a *prima facie* case for their special educational needs to be met.

But the definition, while going much further than previous definitions, is puzzling in a number of respects. It is puzzling that, if the condition is not the result of any known structural brain-defect and is only "probably" due to maturational lag but is cognitive in essence, we still do not know precisely what the nature of the disability is. Again, we are told that the condition is "usually genetically determined" but we are not told how or given any evidence of the genetic mechanism involved. Does the definition perhaps mean that these children have a cognitive condition in that they have a learning difficulty? Does their probable maturational lag mean that the problem is developmental, that is, that their learning difficulty, which "tends to lessen" as they grow older, is developmental? And is their learning difficulty with reading, writing and spelling? If that is the case then, once again, we have a circular definition. Developmental dyslexia means developmental difficulties in learning to read, write and spell. The definition is no better than terms like specific learning difficulties in reading, specific severe reading retardation.

One of the most disappointing aspects of this definition is that, for all the undoubted medical authority of its authorship, it does not give any signs or symptoms by which developmental dyslexia in children may be recognized other than by its initial manifestation as "a difficulty in learning to read". Although elsewhere Critchley insists that "the diagnosis of specific developmental dyslexia is a medical responsibility" and that it must be differentiated from difficulties due to structural brain damage and minimum brain damage, it is not clear how dyslexia itself is diagnosed medically. While he maintains elsewhere that "Dyslexia implies vastly more than a delay in learning to read, which is but the tip of the iceberg," his description of the rest of the iceberg sounds remarkably like reading and spelling difficulties: "The etymology of the term dyslexia expresses admirably a difficulty — not with reading — but in the use of words, how they are identified, what they signify, how they are handled in combination, how they are pronounced, and how they are spelt." If this isn't a reading, writing and spelling difficulty and is more extensive than that, it must constitute a language problem of considerable intellectual proportions.

That we raise these queries about the difficulties surrounding the term and its definitions is of little consequence, perhaps. But it is because of these difficulties, both of the frequently changing definitions and the variety of symptoms which have been from time to time associated with developmental dyslexia, that the British Medical Association has advised doctors that it is not susceptible to medical diagnosis and that the condition should be considered the provenance of educational psychologists. Interestingly enough, Critchley argues strongly in favour of educational treatment as "the rational remedy".

It is hardly surprising that, as long ago as 1968, Ravenette wrote: "Thus the definitions of 'dyslexia' seem to be variations on a physiological theme, each variation being composed by a different specialist . . . The controversy as it stands is futile. It needs to be dropped and a fresh beginning made." But the controversy has not been dropped and the search for new variations on the physiological theme has gone further and further into the mists of speculation and non-science. It is as if researchers and specialists had become fixated upon dyspepsia and devoted years of research to producing more and more reasons for it with more and more sophisticated definitions but refused to admit they were only investigating indigestion — or an attack of the burps.

Frank Smith tried to nail dyslexia down:

> This term is a name, not an explanation. Dyslexia means, quite literally, being unable to read. Children who experience difficulty learning to read are frequently called dyslexic, but their difficulty does not arise because they *are* dyslexic, or because they *have* dyslexia; they are dyslexic because they cannot read. To say that dyslexia is a cause of not being able to read is analagous to saying that lameness is a cause of not being able to walk . . . The cure for dyslexia is to learn to read.

Precisely the same can be said about terms like "specific reading retardation" and "specific learning difficulties in reading" and their supporting definitions and descriptions. All the terms do is to put a

gloss on the fact that some children have reading difficulties without telling us what they are or why they exist. Their spurious use of
"specific" neither determines a species nor is it precise. Suggesting
that a disparity between "intelligence" and reading ability is a
"specific retardation" is as fatuous as talking about "specific
singing retardation" or "specific swimming retardation". If you
have difficulty in singing or swimming that's it. "Specific learning
difficulties in reading" begs the question whether the specificity is
in the learning, in the difficulties or in the reading. All it means is
that a child has difficulties in learning to read and there is no need to
be any more specific than that. What one wants to be specific about
are the children's needs and those aspects of the process of learning
to read in which they need help.

It is when we turn to address those problems that the cat is out of
the bag. The neurologists look at the pathological conditions
of their patients with acquired dyslexia and the children with
reading difficulties and begin wondering what reading is all about.
Critchley analyses the process by starting with the recognition
of individual letters, their orientation, combinations and the
problems of phonics. Nowhere does he begin to conceptualize
reading as anything but going from print to sound, or what used to
be called "barking at print": reading is sounds in print and
learning to read is little more than decoding the alphabetical
symbols. Not surprisingly, with this view of reading, children are
seen to have cognitive difficulties because Critchley himself jumps
the cognitive gap: "Then comes the two-fold task of reading aloud
not only with correct articulation, but also with simultaneous
understanding". In other words, the problem with defining
precisely and specifically what the children's difficulties are is
nothing to do with the children or their difficulties. It is a problem
of defining the process of reading.

Teachers and educational psychologists tend to see the problem
quite differently. They look at all the children who have succeeded
in learning to read successfully despite physical, sensory, intellectual and environmental difficulties and at those who can't read
but should, and wonder what reading is all about. They see it as a
complex of skills and subskills which somehow children succeed in
getting all together and making sense. They are amazed that
children can do it. As the American psychologist Neisser observed:
"We may not understand reading until we understand thought

itself". But they know that different children somehow learn to read at different times at different rates and in different ways. They are not surprised that some children find it difficult. *They see reading as getting sense or meaning from print as the first, not the last step. They start with the cognitive gap. The fact that some of them get stuck in it and start to worry about things like "intelligence", or what they now prefer to call achievement on tests of ability and performance, may well lead them into the miasmas of psychological speculation where they meet up with the neurologists coming back.* Increasingly, however, more and more of them are addressing themselves to the fact that what needs tackling is a deeper understanding of the reading process and how children may be helped to learn.

What to do with the word "dyslexia"

There is no doubt that some children have difficulties in reading. We have the greatest admiration for all that has been done by neurologists and neuro-psychologists, psychologists and therapists, to investigate, illuminate and ventilate the children's problems. In the process they have introduced their work-horse medical term into the language. It is now simply no more and no less than synonymous with difficulties in reading which is how it was born into our naughty world in all its nakedness. But it has the advantage, when applied to children, or adults that it is now used in common parlance only for those who we think ought to be able to read but can't. We don't say babies are dyslexic although we may say some actresses are. We don't say people who have never been to school and haven't learned to read are dyslexic, we say they are illiterate or semiliterate as the case may be. Use determines meaning and usage has already determined that "dyslexia" and "dyslexic" have entered the language as useful terms of no greater specificity or medical pretension than "dyspepsia" or "dyspeptic". Instead of trying to define them or investigate them in isolation, research must be directed at the processes of learning and the processes of reading as assuredly as our dyspepsia researchers must direct their efforts at the process of digestion. We are reminded of some lines of Ogden Nash which may serve as some solace to those who may regret the demise of dyslexia from medical grace to the market place:

> A good deal of superciliousness
> Is based on biliousness.
> People seem as proud as peacocks
> Of any infirmity, be it hives or dementia praecox.

Children do not need the label of dyslexia. What is needed are more discriminating approaches to meet these children's special educational needs and the needs of all children to realize their right to read. We need to see those needs in the contexts of human diversity, the processes of learning and reading, and the problems of literacy in our societies.

Reading difficulties in the context of adult illiteracy

About two million people or 6% of the adult population are estimated by the Adult Literacy and Basic Skills Unit in England to be functionally illiterate. In the USA the "Survival Literacy Study", conducted for the US National Reading Council in 1970, found that 34% of Americans could not adequately read an application for medical aid, 11% were unable to complete a form for a personal bank loan, and 8% could not complete a request for a driving licence. The concept of functional literacy was first used in Unesco international surveys of reading in 1956. It defines a literate person as one who has acquired the essential knowledge and skills which enable him to engage in all those activities in which literacy is required for effective functioning in his group and community. It is a relative term and can thus be used to describe the minimal level of literacy acceptable in any society. Different societies make different demands for literacy. As societies develop, so the demands for higher levels of literacy increase.

In the highly-developed, complex industrial and multi-ethnic commercial societies of Europe and North America, with their form-filling bureaucracies, the demand is for increasingly higher levels of literacy. In the underdeveloped Third World, the demand is for basic literacy as a prerequisite for social, agricultural, industrial and political development. In Africa, the continent with the highest levels of illiteracy, 98% of the black population is illiterate. In Asia and Pacific Countries, with the exception of Japan, about 55% of the population between 6 and 14 years will grow up illiterate. In China, a quarter of the population between 12 and 45 is

illiterate. Even in some parts of Southern Europe, in rural areas of
Spain, Portugal and Italy, as much as 50% of the population is still
illiterate in that they are below the minimal level of functional
literacy. Throughout the world enormous efforts are being made to
change this situation and to give people the right to read.

Since the setting up of the Adult Illiteracy programme in England
and Wales, 200,000 adults have sought help in basic literacy skills
and currently 80,000 are being helped. Large though these
numbers are, many people consider them but the tip of the iceberg.
Anyone who has worked with adult illiterates knows how much
courage it takes them, after years of subterfuge to hide their sense
of inadequacy and the stigma of being unable to read, just to pick
up a phone and ask for help. Many cannot bring themselves to this
point, and many who do fail to take the next step of going for an
advice interview. Often, as a result, the teachers and volunteers
who run the courses find that their students are not so much the
illiterate as the semi-literate. They can write their own names and
read a little but cannot read a newspaper, complete forms or write
simple letters. They are functionally illiterate but are still not the
complete non-readers or illiterates with whom they originally
thought they would be dealing. However, helping these students
has proved to be a long and demanding process and very different
from the short, sharp mopping-up operation the government
thought it would be a decade ago. It is now recognized that not only
are there more people than was originally thought who are in need
of help with basic literacy skills, but that their needs cannot be
readily met. Moreover, these students are not unintelligent or
incapable of learning and by no means all of them can attribute their
problems to social deprivation or poor schooling. Frequently, there
are a whole variety of factors, such as missed schooling, frequent
school changes, social and emotional factors and an early sense of
failure, which led to an avoidance of reading and to hiding their
difficulties, which may account for their problems. Some people, it
is also argued, are never going to acquire functional literacy simply
by attending ordinary schools and will need continued skilled help
and support well into adult life.

Illiteracy — The size of the problem

At first glance it is surprising that in societies like our own, which have enjoyed or suffered, as the case may be, universal and free education for over a century, we only have "guesstimates" of the numbers of illiterates and semi-literates. One reason for this is the difficulty of defining what the terms mean in any sensible and satisfactory manner. As we have already seen, the concept of "functional literacy" is both a recent one and a relative one. Previously, we have relied in our education systems on reading tests which were ill-conceived and, as the years went by, became more and more out of date, even in the language they used. They failed to reflect society's demands for higher levels of literacy or changes in our understanding of the reading process. Only in the past decade has it been widely recognized that the available statistical evidence of levels of literacy was suspect. Not only were the tests used a reflection of a narrow and inadequate concept of reading, but they failed to distinguish between the most able readers at the top of the scales and failed to give any meaningful description of the levels of skill attained by the least able readers. As the Bullock Report of the Committee of Inquiry appointed by Mrs Thatcher, then Secretary of State for Education and Science in 1972, *A Language for Life*, makes clear, "All estimates of the number of illiterates and semi-literates in the population must therefore be hedged about with reservations. Nevertheless, it is obvious that although they represent a small percentage of the total population their numbers are considerable." The best the Report could do was cite the evidence of national surveys of reading in schools which found that 3.18% of 15-year-olds in England and Wales, or nearly 15,000 pupils aged 15 years, read above the 7-year-old level but below the 9-year-old level. Illiteracy was defined as reading below the 7-year-old level, and 0.42% of 11-year-old pupils were illiterate. Of the 11-year-olds, 15.1% were semi-literate, that is, were reading below the 9-year-old level.

At first glance these disconcerting figures appear to be telling us something significant about various levels of literacy. In fact, they tell us remarkably little and beg more questions than they answer. The reading test used was a test of silent sentence comprehension. All the pupils were required to do was read through a list of sixty sentences arranged in order of difficulty. Each sentence had three words in brackets and the correct one had to be underlined for the pupils to score. For example:

They went to the shop to (say, buy, look) some bread.

When the statistics tell us that some pupils aged 15 only read at the 9-year-old level this simply means that they got right only the same *total* number of sentences as the average 9-year-old. The "levels" or reading ages tell us nothing about the skills acquired or the characteristics of the reading abilities of the pupils. The underlying assumption behind this method of assigning levels of reading or reading ages is that reading ability can be divided up into equal units of level of difficulty and that these levels can be related to equal units of age in years and months. As the Bullock Report pointed out, "there are no grounds whatever for supposing that reading progress is a linear process of this kind, and indeed there is evidence to the contrary".

The tests did not test the accuracy or speed of reading, did not test the ability to read a paragraph and recall or make inferences from the information it contained, nor did the tests examine the ability of pupils to cope with different levels of difficulty in their reading in the various subjects of the school curriculum. In view of this limited sampling of reading ability it might have been expected that considerable stringency would have been applied in determining what constituted illiteracy and semi-literacy. However, as we have seen, 15-year-olds who read at the 7 to 9-year-old level on the test are considered semi-literate. If we therefore accept that 15-year-olds who read at the 10-year-old level are backward in reading but, nonetheless, literate, it is clear that we have a very limited view of what constitutes literacy. In terms of this test it means no more than reading a couple of dozen simple sentences.

In fact, in our society, functional literacy, in any meaningful and practical sense, requires at least the ability of the average 15-year-old if we are to read fluently and with insight and understanding over a wide range of subjects from income-tax and insurance forms to notices and newspapers. But, unfortunately, this test even failed to examine how well 15-year-olds could read. The test was not only 16 years old, and failed to reflect change in the usage of language and in our understanding of the reading process, it was found to be too easy for more able 15-year-olds to show their ability. Even on silent comprehension reading, the results do not tell us what abilities the average 15-year-olds have: there is just a lot of them all lumped together indiscriminately at the top.

The results of this survey have been subject to quite sophisticated statistical analysis and are frequently cited and discussed. Clearly, it is important that we know what is going on in our schools and plan accordingly in such a vital area as literacy. Clearly, we need to understand why so many 11-year-olds enter secondary education unable to read adequately. But no matter how sophisticated the statistics, the results of such tests as this will never tell us. It is strange that societies which value literacy so highly study the resource of their children's abilities so crudely. It is very much as if we observed matter through broken bottle bottoms and thought that, by subjecting our observations to the rigours of quantum mechanics, we could build an atomic-power station.

Hidden behind the inadequacy of surveys such as this and their busy statistics is the stark fact that many thousands of children are struggling through school barely able to read, many thousands in our socially and culturally disadvantaged areas are severely retarded in reading, and each year thousands of pupils leave school to join the millions who are functionally illiterate. We may need better test instruments of reading ability, but we need first higher standards of literacy and more comprehensive and discriminating ways of teaching reading. Hidden, too, are those children with special and specific needs for help in learning to read.

The incidence of dyslexia in children

In the absence of adequate measures of literacy and of agreed criteria by which children's performance may be assessed, it is not surprising to find that both nationally and internationally there are no reliable figures for the incidence of dyslexia. The problem is exacerbated by the absence of agreement as to how dyslexia in children is described qualitatively and quantitatively: What are their specific reading difficulties? What degrees of severity distinguish dyslexic children from poor, slow, backward and normal readers?

There is no figure for the incidence of dyslexia, only a range of figures. The range extends from less than 1% to more than 25%. Figures vary from country to country, from area to area, from specialist to specialist, and from researcher to researcher. The figures depend, in other words, on where one looks, how one looks, what one is looking for, and on who is looking. In this state of affairs it is idle to speculate or to play the numbers game. Nor should one be surprised. What would we expect to be the answer if we asked for the incidence of dyspepsia nationally and internationally? Would we ask the manufacturers of bismuth? What burp-quotient would we use?

However, in the UK we know from the Isle of Wight study, to which we have already referred, that about 4% of the children were found to be severely retarded in reading. At age 11 years, their reading was 28 months below the levels of their ability or IQ. When they were retested at 14 years, the majority had made little progress and were lagging even further behind their peers. When the same or similar criteria have been applied in a similar area, very similar figures of incidence of "severe specific reading retardation" have been reported. Much higher incidence has been found in poor socio-economic areas. By any standards such children are severely retarded and it has been argued that the criteria are too stringent.

It might be thought that in Scandinavian countries, which do not suffer the vagaries of English spelling, the incidence of dyslexia or severe reading difficulties would be markedly lower than in English-speaking countries. But incidence figures of 5% are common.

Only Japan reports a figure of just under 1% for severe reading difficulties. This is surprising, in that Japanese uses a combination of symbols in its print and writing. One set of symbols represents phonetic syllables. These are phonetically consistent: that is, they always represent the same sound. The other set of symbols is derived from Chinese ideograms or logograms. These give the reader clues to the meaning of the words. Only by the end of their school careers do most children master the minimum 2,000 ideographic characters. Despite this demanding and complex system, it appears that the ideograms help both some patients with acquired dyslexia and children learning to read to make sense of the print. If this is so, it suggests that, instead of looking for the incidence of dyslexia or for more discriminating descriptions and definitions, we should be looking more searchingly at what is involved in the process of reading and of how we teach children to read. In English-speaking countries we still seem to be having difficulty in helping some children and in developing adequate levels of literacy generally, with our 26 letter alphabet and 44 phonemes.

Criteria for literacy

One of the most satisfactory methods of assessing young children's reading ability is by finding out from their teachers what books they can read. This, in essence, was the method adopted by the National Foundation for Educational Research in the survey of reading abilities of primary school children in Kent as long ago as 1959 and 1966. This found that 18% of 11-year-old children were still virtual non-readers. By using as one of her major sources of information the primers or basal readers read by the younger children, Joyce Morris was able to make a detailed analysis of reading standards and progress. Today many measures are readily available to teachers and researchers to examine what is called the "readability" of texts and it is to be regretted that more has not been done to develop easily administered and more reliable and discerning tests for older pupils who have progressed beyond the primer stages of reading. Such tests would enable a more valid assessment of reading ability to be made throughout the age-ranges. They would be of value both to teachers and to researchers so that children's needs could be assessed and educational planning of provisions nationally, locally and in the schools, addressed to meeting them. What also needs to be done is to establish the criteria by which levels of literacy can be assessed. It is fatuous to talk about "reading ages" when one bright 8-year-old is enjoying *A Thousand and One Dalmatians, Charlie and the Chocolate Factory* and working her way through Jules Verne, while another equally bright and able reader aged 8 years, with the same reading age of 12.9 years on a test, never reads a book or comic and cannot understand her school books. Similarly, quite apart from determining levels of the *use* made of reading by pupils, we need criteria for establishing how well pupils have developed the functional skills of reading for use in lessons, in project work and in homework.

In this connection, in the NFER study of reading progress and attainment in Scotland, Maxwell found that although illiteracy in his terms was at no more than the 1% level, insufficient attention was being given to the reading and understanding of mathematics text books in primary schools and to pupils' abilities in the 11 to 16 age-range in the different subject areas of the curriculum. By establishing criteria of styles or types of reading, this research provides valuable insights into the problems of functional literacy and what needs to be done to develop it. The six styles of reading identified are:

1. Rapid reading for gist of passage;
2. rapid reading for specified information;
3. rapid reading for relevant information;
4. detailed reading to follow instructions;
5. detailed reading to follow argument;
6. reading for appreciation of style.

The conclusion that in the secondary schools studied, "The teaching of functional reading outwith [i.e. "outside of"] English teaching has virtually disappeared, except for some language activities," is supported by the fact that, "Over half of the good readers and three-quarters of the poor readers failed to make any progress in their reading status" after they moved from primary to secondary school.

One of the dangers of complacency is that these low levels of literacy conceal both the complexity of children's needs and the numbers of children with special needs. If levels of reading and methods of teaching reading are assessed by more stringent and searching methods, the needs of children are thrown into sharp relief. The Schools Council Project "Extending Beginning Reading", for example, demonstrated the futility of teachers trying to give individual help to pupils if this, as the research showed, is for no more than an average of 30 seconds at a time. What the children need is: less frequent but much longer, say 15 to 20 minute periods of individual help and attention; opportunities for longer periods of undisturbed silent reading; help and guidance in the development of study skills and the use of books as tools; the diagnosis of their weaknesses which should provide the source and guidance for individual and group correction, rather than the pupils being kept in lock-step with reading primers or basal readers. But this variety of class, group and individual help with reading and its associated skills can only be developed if teachers are concerned to develop effective reading skills and not lulled into a false sense of security by the children's performance on inadequate reading tests. As this research showed, although most of the 7 to 8-year-olds had mastered the mechanics of reading aloud "they were operating only at the level of word recognition" and not using contextual clues. Again, the research shows careful analysis of the kinds of books being read by children, of the miscues the children made and the strategies they used when asked to read a passage from *More About Paddington* the reading level of which had been determined as being at the 9+ level.

Responsibilities for literacy

These two researches demonstrate the degrees of sophistication which needs to be developed before meaningful and significant statements about reading and its assessment can be made. Only when more sophisticated procedures are developed and widely used will we have adequate statistics about the levels of literacy of the pupils in our schools. Only then will we have adequate indicators of the most effective ways by which teachers may raise standards by improving methods of instruction, classroom management and organization. Only then will it be possible to identify, early enough and discretely enough, those children needing special help.

A general concern for literacy is not enough. Generalized conclusions from simplistic tests of word recognition or sentence completion are not enough. If we are really concerned for reading we must look closely at how children read, what they read and the uses they make of reading. As Maxwell concludes his study: "The essence of effective teaching is that the pupils should know what they have to do, should know how to do it, should know when it is done and should know how well it has been done." If this is to be done, then we must have a much deeper and richer understanding of the process of reading. From that model of reading we must identify the levels of mastery or the criterion reference points along the road from wanting to learn to read, to learning to read, and from learning to read just to get the gist of a passage, to reading with enjoyment, discrimination, selective attention, evaluation and appreciation of argument or style. It means understanding, commitment and sensitivity deployed to the continuous development of literacy in all children.

If, for political, social or philosophical reasons, we want children to be educated in our complex and competitive societies in multi-ethnic schools with a broad spectrum of social classes; if we want them educated in mixed-ability classes into which progressively more and more children with physical, sensory, mental, emotional and behavioural difficulties are successfully integrated: then we have a responsibility to provide levels of expertise and resources appropriate to ensure that each child will, nonetheless, realize his or her full potential as a reader. We have the same responsibility if we segregate children culturally, socially, or according to ability or disability. The responsibility, we suggest, cannot be evaded nor can it be placed on the forms of school organization and educational administration. Learning begins at home and is extended in the classroom. The partnership and shared concerns of parents and teachers, sensitive to the demands of society, and working in harmony with one another and with the changing and developing needs of the child are what determine, in the last analysis, levels of literacy. Literacy is not developed by legislation alone.

Levels of literacy are determined by the richness and variety of opportunities to read and by the incentives to develop and use the skills of reading. An observer in Northumberland recorded that in almost every village children were found able to read and write at a very early age. That was in 1839, well before the Elementary Education Act of 1870. An Italian physician visiting the United States in the 1810s, recorded that "these people are not quasi-barbarians; one does not find here the ignorant peasantry that one finds in our country". In the last quarter of a century, from the 1950s to 1976, world illiteracy fell from 50% to 30%. In Cuba and Nicaragua short but highly intensive programmes have achieved spectacular improvements in levels of literacy in less than a year. In Jamaica and Tanzania, steady and substantial progress has been made over recent years. In Britain and North America, where mass literacy is a right and not a privilege, the concern to raise basic levels of functional literacy has shown steady progress in our schools and has already gone some way to meeting the needs of thousands of adults. But we cannot escape the conclusion that far too many children leave our schools without functional literacy at a level commensurate with the demands society makes upon them, and that many more are insecure in those skills of reading and writing of which they are capable. And among these children are some whose difficulties often appear deep-seated, profound and intractable. *It is our belief that, whether children's difficulties are the result of environmental factors or of factors within the child, their needs will only be met by appropriate opportunities and appropriate incentives — including the motivation to read.* These opportunities and incentives can only be provided if we understand the complexities of the process of reading.

CHAPTER 3

The Process of Reading

"He has only half learned the art of reading who has not added to it the even more refined accomplishments of skipping and skimming." Lord Arthur Balfour

The use of language is a natural attribute of man. The ability to read, however, is an acquired skill. We are born with the innate propensity to develop understanding and use of language and all that is necessary is that we should be exposed to it in a social setting. By about the age of two we understand and use language. Whether our mother tongue is Chinese, Arabic or English makes no difference. It is rather like our ability to walk. Whether we are natural crawlers or bottom-shufflers makes no difference, nor does it matter whether we are wrapped up and tied to our mothers' backs for the first year or put in baby-walkers, we will learn to walk upright when we are ready. Learning to read is more like learning to ride a bike, it is a complex and acquired skill.

Getting bike-borne and print-borne

The sequence in which we learn the skills of riding and reading is similar. First we learn to walk and then we have to learn the special skills involved in riding a bike; we learn language and then we have to learn the special skills of reading. There are other similarities. We first have to have a good idea of what it means to ride: we need to have a model of the accomplishment and to want desperately to

master it. In the same way, we must know what it means to be able
to read and be convinced that it is a worthwhile ability which we
want to master and enjoy.

Both skills can be analysed in term of subskills, but the essential
knack is to learn to get them all together. Being able to steer and to
pedal is not enough to enable us to ride. Knowing our letters and
how to look at them from left to right is not the same as being able to
read. No matter how well we may know all the separate subskills,
until we can perform them all simultaneously we will fall off the
bike or fail at reading. As if this were not daunting enough, all the
subskills have to become automatized. The child who must look
down all the time to make sure the feet are on the pedals is riding
for a fall as assuredly as the child who cannot see the words for the
letters or the sense for the words. Riding a bike and reading a book
demand that all the subskills and their co-ordination are so automatized that we scarcely need to think of them and can concentrate
not on what we are doing but upon where we are going.

The physics and neuro-physiology of riding a bike are so complex that no one with an iota of common sense would think of
exposing a child to the process! In spite of this, parents sit their
children on bikes, support them, help them to get going and utter
words of advice. They begin by doing most of the work themselves
but, little by little, as the children grow in skill and confidence, the
parents do less and less and even let go altogether for brief
moments. Then, suddenly, the kids get the knack and they are
bike-borne. Some practice and a few trial runs, and they have
acquired a skill which they will be able to develop and enjoy for the
rest of their lives. Some children will go on to road-racing, some to
track events, some will travel far and wide, and others will be
content to use it just to get around the neighbourhood.

Learning to read follows a similar course. We still don't understand the neuro-psychology involved, but all that is needed, once
children have a model of the activity and want to master it for
themselves, is to have a parent or someone else they can trust to
give them a start by reading to them, reading with them and for
them, and gradually letting them do a little bit on their own. As
they grow in skill and confidence they will get the subskills more
and more together, more and more automatized, until one day they
have the knack and they are print-borne. Almost from the beginning of print, once the secret got out of the hands of elites, this

is what parents and teachers have done. When the Bible was the only book a family possessed the children used it as their primer or basal reader. Learning to read is a much less threatening and physically less hazardous process than learning to ride a bike, of course. No one has fallen off a book and broken an arm. It is also a process which, unlike riding a bike, can be done in reverse: long before children have mastered the decoding of print they can be learning many of the subskills involved by writing, by encoding language in writing. This again is something which parents help their children to do. They may well begin by teaching the children to write their own names and, by so doing, teach them one of the secrets of print and the key to the whole process of reading. That key is that print isn't speech.

The gulf between spoken and printed language

A great white gulf separates reading from spoken language. Speech proceeds in time and we catch it as it flows by. It flows on, often without appreciable pauses between words and sometimes with distinct pauses within words. This is something of which we are often unaware until we listen to a foreign language with which we are completely unfamiliar. But even when we attend to a foreign language, we may grasp some meaning from the speaker's expression, from the way the voice rises and falls. The cadence and expression may carry more meaning than the words we hear in our own language. "I'd rather you didn't do that", can be accented on each of its words and convey a variety of meanings, including its opposite! It isn't what we say, but the way that we say it which is an essential ingredient of spoken language and conveys so much of the message. This component of spoken language is almost completely lacking in print. Even with dramatic writing the producer and actors can only attempt a feasible approximation to what the dramatist intended his dialogue to sound like.

Print proceeds linearly and, in our culture, from left to right. Language is divided up into words and many of the words which are elided in speech, the "little words" of language such as *the*, *it* or *be*, assume a new significance. We put white spaces between the words, aconventionwhichmakesfor clarity, perhaps, but which didn't trouble mediaeval monks reading the manuscripts from which spaces were absent because often they knew by heart what they were reading.

We put spaces between the letters, too, but don't do this in cursive writing. These conventions of print are something we have to learn. But there is nothing predestined about them. Arabic and Hebrew go from right to left. At one time Ancient Greek followed the plough and went along one line from left to right and back along the next line from right to left. For centuries Chinese and Japanese went from bottom to top of the page. The human brain is perfectly able to adapt to a variety of conventions because human brains devised them. The diversity of codes man has devised for recording his thoughts demonstrates that it is not speech which is being recorded. Ancient Egyptians used pictograms and Chinese and Japanese use ideograms or symbols. The fact that we use alphabetic symbols for sounds should not blind us to the fact that it is not sounds that we get from the messages of print but meaning. The Chinese get the meaning first and then have to put their own sounds, according to where they live, to the meaning. We have to get the meaning from the message before we can determine the sounds, too, in many instances. *Reading*, for instance, may be an activity or a place. How we say *the* depends upon whether it is followed by a vowel or a consonant. In spoken language the meaning is the message: in retrieving written language we must find its meaning before we can reconstitute its sound.

Unfortunately, that gulf is widened by the fact that, in attending to speech, we are given so many more additional cues to the speaker's meaning. Not only are we helped by how he expresses himself, we are helped by the expression on his face, which may be at variance with the words and phrases he is using. We are also helped by the situation in which we are a part. The speaker gestures as he speaks, points or glances towards whatever or at whomsoever he is making reference. Thus, he may not name a person or object but use a gesture and a pronoun and his meaning is quite clear. Spoken language is in a situation in which we are participants and in which there are mutually understood referents. But when listening to speech on a radio, unless we are cued into the situation and know whether we are listening to, say, the news or a talk, a play or a documentary, we may be unsure of its meaning and significance. The people who rushed out into the streets of American cities when they heard Orson Welles' broadcast of *War of the Worlds* thought they were listening to a news broadcast. Such misunderstandings are rare in spoken language because of all the cues we have to meaning. But these cues are largely lacking in written langauge. This is demonstrated by the immediacy of television versions of novels which in their opening shots can present characters and establish their ages, mannerisms, situations and historical period, facts and details which took, perhaps, chapters in the original. The demands made upon the reader, therefore, are considerable, for the text must establish the situation in which the reader is not yet a participant and gradually involve him until he does, in fact, participate. Notice how one popular children's book begins:

> One thing was certain, that the *white* kitten had nothing to do with it — it was the black kitten's fault entirely.

The tone is conversational, an attempt is even made to introduce emphasis by the convention of using italics, but only in the next sentence will the reader find out what *it* was, which happens to be mischief. What the mischief was is only revealed in the third paragraph. The same writer was well aware of the problem. He begins another book like this:

> Alice was beginning to get very tired of sitting by her sister on the bank, and of having nothing to do: once or twice she had peeped into the book her sister was reading, but it had no pictures or conversations in it, "and what is the use of a book," thought Alice, "without pictures or conversations?"

Pictures in books and comics, conversation, whether in inverted commas or in captions or bubbles, provide children with the situational cues to understanding which otherwise have to be embedded in pages of print. The language of books is language which must, perforce, be more particular and explicit than the language of everyday speech. In making meaning clear, language in print is itself a convention with which the reader must come to terms. We can only introduce children to this language by reading it to them so that they have acquired the language before they in turn will one day read it with enjoyment and understanding. That is far more important than teaching them to read by looking at the letters or making their sounds.

What divides spoken language from print in the final analysis makes little difference. Whether we hear the word "Stop!", hear a fire-engine approaching, see the red light or see the word "Stop!", what is important is that we understand their meanings. What unites spoken language and printed language is their meaning. What is on the surface, whether it be sound or symbol, must first be attended to, then be placed in its situation or context before, aided by our memory, we can attribute the appropriate significance or meaning. The sound "Look!" means nothing unless we know where to look. What we see when we look will determine the meaning of the speaker's exclamation and we will share his pleasure or horror. Finding out what is meant by "Look!" upon the printed page depends upon our memory of what we have already read and upon our ability to hold it in memory until we have read what follows. We must go from the surface structure of print to the deep structure of meaning. That, in the final analysis, is the extent of the gulf between print and speech: they meet only in the depths of memory and of meaning.

Reading isn't only reading words

To appreciate fully the problem of learning to read we need to look beyond words. In particular it is useful to look at other forms of reading in which we interpret visual information. The earliest activities of man, food gathering and hunting, involved reading the prints of animals, the signs of changing weather and climate, and the recognition of food-bearing grasses and plants. We remember Stuart whose teacher assured us he couldn't read because he couldn't interpret visual information. We asked Stuart to look out of the window and tell us what he could see. "Grass," said Stuart. "What can you tell us about the grass?" we asked. "It's been cut," answered Stuart promptly, thereby demonstrating that he could both discern the stripes of the mower and interpret visual information into language.

When man began recording information he began by imitating the same forms of recording he had observed around him. He made his marks on trees, on clay and rock, he put knots in strips of hide. Knowing what the marks meant when he made them, he had no difficulty in recalling them later. They served as aids to memory.

Children make pictures which, in their early years, we cannot interpret but they can tell us about. Children, long before they learn to use Arabic numbers, make strokes and each stroke stands for the thing they have counted. They are learning that each stroke stands for a thing, that there is a one-to-one correspondence.

Early writing began as pictures or pictograms. Our world is still full of them. Jenny, who couldn't read, knew all the common roadsigns for humped-back bridges, crossroads, junctions and Z-bends. Recognition of signs and symbols is a vital stage in learning and in learning to read. But some children have never had their attention drawn to them. Other children have learned them but no one has ever bothered to find out whether or not they know them. Some children who have severe learning difficulties can be greatly helped in developing perception and in learning to read by introducing them to rebuses or pictograms for common objects like house ⌂ and ball ◐   . The Peabody Rebus Program is an excellent development of this. It has helped many children to learn to learn and to develop language and communication skills. Some, who otherwise wouldn't, have gone on from reading rebuses to reading print.

One form of reading is rarely considered but provides an illuminating parallel with reading print. Many of us who find it difficult to appreciate children's reading difficulties find it a salutory experience to study a musical score. What is the relationship between the black dots and the sounds we hear? How competent are we in taking up a full orchestral score and, simply by reading it, hearing in our minds something of the music? And how do we account for the fact that Jimmie, who can't read books and is cross-lateral, that is, in his case right-handed but left-eyed, reads music which he plays with both hands on the piano? Is it an adequate explanation of his difficulties with print to argue that they are caused by cross-laterality or the inability to associate what he sees with what he hears? Perhaps Jimmie's difficulties lie in the fact that a different part of his brain is involved in language processing from the bit involved in hearing and processing music. But when we ask Jimmie what key he is playing in he looks at the key signature and tells us "the key of G". It may be that Jimmie's difficulties have arisen because, in trying to teach him to read, we have put him in the same position as many adults are placed when confronted with a musical score.

We take reading print so much for granted that parents and teachers who have spent a dozen or more years being educated assume that it is a natural skill which anyone with an IQ of 75 or over can pick up with a modicum of help and encouragement. We recall a College of Education which introduced a compulsory unit in its curriculum for all students in the "Teaching of Reading". This produced loud protests from all the students training to teach the 11–16 age group: teaching reading wasn't for them, they were training to teach English, History, Geography, Mathematics and the Sciences, etc. The unit was eventually dropped because of their protests. No doubt these students, who are now distinguishing themselves in their subject specialisms in our schools, inveigh against their pupils who have difficulties in writing up their notes, completing their assignments, reading their textbooks and writing their essays. But the point we wish to make is a different one. How many of them can read $E = mc^2$, or $N_2 + 3H_2 = 2NH_3$, or distinguish between $\propto$ and ∞? In other words, reading includes understanding relativity, ammonia and the difference between "being proportional to" and infinity. Using symbols and conventional signs, whether in chemistry, circuitry or maps, is all a part of reading. But unless we know and understand what the symbols represent and the concepts or ideas they embody, we cannot read them. To help children to learn to read we have to have the insight and the humility to recognize that the skill we take so much for granted is highly complex and not a simple matter of letter recognition but one of gaining meaning and understanding.

The reader who is in any doubt about the importance of meaning in reading is invited to try this little test. Below are ten words selected from Hunter Diack's Standard Literacy Tests. For how many of them can you confidently give a meaning?

aboulia	noumenon
antonomasia	ortolan
chalybeate	pulvinate
dortour	tanagra
grallatorial	velleity

Perhaps readers who get "tied up" saying some of them are "appreciably handicapped by dyslexia" or are insecure in phonic skills and left to right lateral scanning. We suspect, however, that whether or not readers can say the words, they will have had difficulty in giving a meaning to some of them. As the words are from the highest level of Diack's Tests, readers who know them all can be assumed to have a vocabulary of 36,000 words, approximately. As Diack suggests that a vocabulary of about 23,000 words is a minimum for university graduates, however, readers who do not know the meanings of any of them may relax and carry on reading. We trust, however, that we have made the point that reading is a complex skill of gaining meaning and understanding and that it is one which we are continuously learning — by reading.

The surface structure of print

The linearly arranged letters of print are our cues to the meaning of the message. A great deal has been written about the complexity of the rules which bind letters together and about the variety of sounds that each letter or combination of letters may make. The Bullock Report on the teaching of reading in schools, *A Language for Life*, wittily invented the word "calmbost", a phonic substitution of the sounds in the word "chemist" by spellings from other words (such as *c* as in *c*andle, *a* as in m*a*ny), in order to give "some impression of the kind of problem that confronts a child when he has to combine graphemes and phonemes in a phonic attack on an unfamiliar word". It pointed out that in 6,092 two-syllable words in the comprehension vocabularies of 6 to 9-year-old children, researchers had found 211 different spellings for the same sounds which required 166 rules to govern their use. The Report went on to point out that, "The idea that at this level reading consists of matching sounds and symbols in some simple way is therefore quite untenable". The observation would be more accurate if "at this level" were omitted: how do we say "aleatory" and what is the rule for spelling "benefiting"? It is far better to look at reading without bothering about the spelling if one wants to understand the process, we suggest.

Let us imagine that, in these days of mass unemployment, a bright, black, left-handed youth, Jeff, lands a job as a copy typist. Comes the day when the boss's secretary is away and he calls in our bright lad to "take down a letter". Realizing that it is a case of sink or swim, Jeff suppresses the cry of "I don't do shorthand!", takes up pencil and pad and writes, as his boss dictates:

> D.s: Thk u fr yr lttr f 21 S nqrg f w cn spply u wth th gds lstd n yr ordr by 10 N. I m plsd t nfrm u tht I'v tdy md rrngmts w r Trnspt Mgr & u cn xpct dlvry M mrng, 7 N. I trst th wl b cnvt. Thk u fr yr ordr wh wl ctnu to rcv m prsnl attn.
> Yrs f

The boss is impressed with the letter when he signs the typed copy. Being bright, too, he cuts his secretary's dictation load by scribbling comments on letters, such as "Say yes — 15 Dec" and "No — regret no credit", in the certain knowledge that Jeff will write the appropriate letters. Jeff's "shorthand" serves to demonstrate that we can understand an enormous amount of language with the minimum of cues from the spelling.

The boss's "comments" show that a few words can convey the meaning of a long and possibly linguistically complex message. In both cases, of course, we are helped by understanding the situation. This, too, helps us to predict.

The redundancy of print

In other words, the surface structure of print is highly redundant and the reason we can read it so quickly is that we only need minimal clues to get the meaning and to predict what comes next. We are aided in this not only by our knowledge of the situation but also by the frequency with which letters occur in print, and by the frequency with which words follow one another. "Once upon . . ." is all we need to see in order to predict the next likely five words, "a time there was a" at the beginning of a story. It is rare in books about reading and the graphemes, or printed clusters of letters, and the phonemes, or sounds, they represent, to find any recognition of either the basic consistency of the alphabet or the frequency of letters and letter-strings. Instead of worrying about alternative spellings and rules it is far more valuable to recognize that letter frequency in effect reduces the load we must carry in our memories at any one time. Thus, E is the most frequently recurring letter in English. Vowels account for about 40% of all texts and, apart from I and A, which serve as words, carry little meaning and usually have to be ignored or guessed. As the 'shorthand' letter demonstrated, we can manage reasonably well without them. The nine most frequently occurring letters E T A O N R I S H, make up 70% of text. Fifty per cent of words begin with T A O S or W, and 50% end with E S D or T. Similarly, the most common two-letter words are TO IN IS IT BE AS AT SO WE HE BY OR, and the most common three-letter words are THE AND FOR ARE BUT NOT YOU ALL ANY CAN. The most common four-letter words are THAT WITH HAVE THIS WILL YOUR FROM THEY KNOW WANT.

In addition to this high redundancy and high frequency of print, we are also aided in our reading by our knowledge of language which enables us to predict the structure or syntax from a very few cues. As we have seen, language in print is more precise and grammatical than speech but still follows the same basic structural rules. Familiarity with spoken language and its syntax, which is thoroughly established in most children by the age of 4 years, aided by familiarity with written language, through listening to adults and others reading to them, equips most children with the ability to predict what *may* come next in print. Clearly, sentences which begin in the same way are likely to be constructed in the same way. "When he. . . .", "Why do. . . ?", "Although. . . .", "All of a . . .", "After she. . . ." all signal a limited range of options as to what structures can follow. Children have this ability, often from a very early age, which can be annoying should we pause for dramatic effect and they blurt out the punch line. Children of six or seven who are of average ability but cannot guess what comes next have usually been badly taught and are fixated on the print. They are looking at the wrong cues. When we read we do not notice the minor variations of vowel sounds any more than we notice them when we are speaking.

> One of these people on the quay seized the key to the green bathing machine and gave it to the chief officer who threw it in the sea.

That sentence contains seven different ways of spelling the "ee" sound, a fact which troubles no one. We do not confuse "see" with "sea", nor "key" with "quay", when we hear them and there is no reason why they should cause us difficulty when their spelling carefully distinguishes them for us.

Patterns of print and language

Another aid to reading is provided by the pattern both of print and of language. The following question of simple everyday words, from which the familiar patterning has been removed, is almost impossible to decipher:

WH ER EW ER EW EW HE NT HE YW ER ET HE RE?

Deprived of the pattern of words and spaces and of the ascenders and descenders of print we are deprived of the pattern of the familiar words, "Where were we when they were there?" Although we are unable to use the rise and fall of the human voice in processing print, we are able to use the rise and fall of letter shapes and the spacing of short and long words as we scan from left to right. Together with the patterns of familiar clusters of letters and familiar groupings of words in patterns of sense, the patterns of print are decoded into meaning. Some of the letter patterns, moreover, are not phonemes but meaningful units, or morphemes, which we recognize immediately. *Un-, im-, tri-, -ly, -ness, -ous, -ician* or *-ic* are common morphemes. They may help us through a sentence in unfamiliar language the meaning of which may be obscure even if we follow the teachers' instructions to "make the sounds and build the words":

> It will present as central blindness if the visual cortex is affected or as total, homonymous or partial quadratic hemianopia if the lesion is in one occipital region.

But if we don't know what it means before we read a sentence such as that, reading it aloud will make the meaning no clearer. Getting beyond the print to the deep structure of meaning depends on what we bring with us, on the knowledge we have, on our understanding, our imagination and, above all, upon our consciousness of language.

Reading is, then, an acquired skill in which we use a variety of cues to get meaning from the print we scan. As in listening to spoken language, we have to learn to attend to the most significant cues. Just as in listening we can focus our attention so that we can follow a conversation being carried on at the other side of noisy room, so in reading we can focus our attention upon those features of print which will help us to predict or guess its meaning. In scanning down the page of a telephone directory for the name we want, our attention may be focused on the most significant feature of that name, its length, its initial letters or its ending. In reading a sentence we may scan quickly to its end or seek the word we anticipate will complete the sense. A book on a subject with which we are thoroughly familiar, may be read more quickly than the instruction manual for repairing a piece of apparatus with which we are unfamiliar. In this selective attention we are participants in the act of retrieving from print the information and meaning we need or wish to enjoy. We are helped by the surface structure of print which, as we have seen, is highly redundant, highly pre-dictable, patterned and, usually, merely encodes the language we already know.

Models of the reading process

The phonic model

The simplest model of reading may be represented as:

$$\boxed{\text{LETTERS} \rightarrow \text{SOUNDS} \rightarrow \text{WORDS}}$$

It looks the simplest model and although it is the earliest and most primitive model it is one which is frequently used in the teaching of beginning and remedial reading. It is concerned more with what goes on in front of the eyes than behind them, however, and is fraught with difficulties. Some years ago attempts were made to reduce the difficulties of having only 26 letters which are variously combined to make the 44 phonemes, or sound units, of English, by having a phonetically consistent alphabet. This is called the initial teaching alphabet, i.t.a., which certainly makes the early stages of reading and writing easier. As it was new to both children and teachers it also had the in-built advantage of having to be taught thoroughly. So much so that some parents in the North of England complained that their children were "talking posh" when they adopted the long Southern English "a" sound in their everyday speech. However, its use not only entailed using books printed in the alphabet, it also meant that, once the children were reading and writing it, they had to transfer to ordinary print and writing, which was dubbed t.o. or traditional orthography. Of course another difficulty remained unsolved: building up the sounds, no matter how easy we may make that for children, still leaves them with the problems of knowing how to break up the words into syllables (syl-lab-les?) and of recombining them into words. This problem would have been identified if a close look had first been taken at children learning to read in countries which already have phonetically consistent alphabets such as Finland or Czecho-slovakia. Phonetic consistency also has the disadvantage in English of removing the clues to the meanings of words we have embodied in the language from Greek, Latin, Low German, Norman French and virtually every literate and non-literate culture in the world.

Apart from the difficulties of going from letters to sounds to words the model is inadequate in that it fails to account for all the work that has to be done by memory before the words can have meaning. As we have already seen, meaning only gradually un-coils as we scan the lines. The following sentence illustrates the problem:

> The bat in the bag,
> with the stumps,
> gloves and ball,
> was fast asleep.

Only the last word gives us the vital cue that the "bat" is a mammal. However, although the model is crude, so simple is the process of learning to read for the vast majority of children, that teaching methods which are based on it have succeeded with millions of children. It is also true to say that this model, because of its inadequacy, accounts for the many difficulties encountered by children and their teachers. The complexity of the relationships between print and sound is such that the more thoroughly children master simple letter–sound associations the more they must unlearn as they proceed. It is easy enough to begin with "The cat sat on the mat" and to go on to "The tan man ran from the van to the can", but a long, hard and confusing road to being able to cope with, say, a simple notice like, "Danger — No Bathing At High Tide".

To overcome the problem of the various alternative sounds made by common digraphs, pairs of letters such as *ee, ea, oa,* or *ue,* less extreme measures than i.t.a. have been tried. Colour-coding and putting marks to indicate short or long sounds, called diacritic marks, have been used. These certainly reduce some of the confusion but also have the disadvantage of adding yet more to what the child must remember about the shapes and sounds and of diverting attention away from the meaning. Again, of course, given an enthusiastic and strongly motivating teacher who reads aloud to her children and who uses these devices in the context of many other language activities, colour-coding or diactrics may well help children to "crack the code".

Another problem with this model is that it has to come to terms with all the frequently recurring words which don't readily build or blend. Words like *of, was, all, are, one, they, about* and *their,* occur in all texts at the simplest level. These words are frequently taught separately as a "sight vocabulary". For the learner reader the difficulty is, of course, one of remembering what to build and what to recognize on sight, while for the teacher the problem is to determine whether to teach an ever-growing "sight vocabulary" or progressively more complex sounding strategies to encompass words like *garage, people, colonel, chassis or brooch.*

One variation on the model has been to teach the sounds in "phonic words". Instead of learning to split words up into their graphemic–phonemic bits and blend and build them together, as in "thr/oa/t", the child is introduced to words like "*coat*" and "*boat*", which contain common phonemes or sound units. This certainly has the advantage of focusing attention on the word as a meaningful unit. It also overcomes another problem inherent in the phonic approach, that of what is called vocabulary control. If children are to be introduced first to simple and then to increasingly more complex graphemes and phonemes, then it follows that the text must be carefully controlled to provide both frequent repetition and the gradual introduction of new "rules" in words which contain them. The Letters–Sounds–Words model, for all its simplicity, concentrates on the surface structure of print and, in so doing, becomes progressively more complex. Of course, letters and groups of letters in English make approximations to sounds and, of course, recognition of the fact that they sequence from left to right is a component in learning to read. But the simple skill is, in fact, a galaxy of subskills. Letter shapes, letter groups or clusters, blends (*th, str-, -ing*), vowel digraphs (*oo, ea*), syllables and building or synthesizing them together, must all be learned. The model is inadequate because it fails to embody the meaningful and structural, syntactical components of language, ignores the predictive and cognitive aspects of reading and fails to account for the importance of memory in the reading process.

Look-and-Say and Sentence Models

In complete contrast to a phonic subskills model Look-and-Say postulates that all that is necessary is for children to be exposed to simple texts and they will rapidly become familiar with the frequently repeated words. The Sentence Model emphasizes that it is the sentence, rather than the word, which is the meaningful unit of sense and that by reading simple texts of simple words in simple sentences children will learn to read. Advocates of this model frequently discouraged sounding and building and believed that the children would respond to graphic shapes of words in the same way as they responded to the sounds they heard. The model was convincingly simple because it appeared to contain the kernel of linguistic sense: children are familiar with language as speech, therefore, all that is necessary is to expose them to language in print. To do this it was only necessary to provide attractive series of books with progressively more demanding texts. As both approaches had to put the words in sentences the differences between them may be conveniently considered as subsumed under the model of "reading for meaning".

By the use of flash-cards and captioned pictures the children were first introduced to the words or sentences they would meet in their primers or basal readers. Reading round the class and reading in groups from the reading schemes were common developments. The approach is particularly successful in countries with phonetically consistent alphabets and with able children in English-speaking countries, particularly if they are familiar with the kind of language used in the books. It is much less successful with linguistically and socially deprived children. Some teachers believed that it was only necessary to surround children with books and they would learn to read, presumably by a process of osmosis. This belief is not completely dead.

However, children who are used to being read to and are pre-pared to guess, frequently find that this is the only introduction they need to reading. If they have good memories for the shapes of letters and words, too, they will soon master many of the irregularities of spelling, of phonemic–graphemic correspondence, and be prepared to attack unfamiliar words which, they will know, have got to make sense in the context of the sentence and story. A Unesco international survey found that the sentence method was used in 46 countries in 1956 and the First Report of the National Child Development Study, *11,000 Seven Year Olds,* in 1966, found that nearly 70% of teachers interviewed did not use a "phonic" method in the initial stages of teaching reading and were using Look-and-Say or Sentence Methods. In fact, many millions of children throughout the world were being introduced to reading using this "reading for meaning" approach and for many millions of children it is still the main method.

However, many children in England and North America failed to learn adequately by the method and there was considerable public concern about levels of literacy and professional controversy which split teachers into two camps, the "phonic" and "whole word or Sentence Method" protagonists. It was quite common by the 1960s to find newly-qualified teachers, apprised of the controversy during their training, claiming to use a "mixed method" approach by combining features of both methods. Many children were introduced to reading by "reading for meaning" and were not introduced to phonics until they were 7 plus. In many instances this meant, in effect, that they received no instruction in reading until they were over 7 years of age. This was because their failure to respond to Look-and-Say or Sentence Methods was attributed to the fact that they were not "reading ready". The doctrine of reading readiness was remotely derived from developmental psychology but had no basis in any neurological or psychological factors which could be measured or observed other than that the children could or could not learn to read. It was a comforting doctrine for many teachers and a worrying one for many parents who were assured that all would be well when their children were "reading ready". It was an alarming doctrine for many education authorities and schools which had to introduce crash programmes to teach large numbers of 7 and 8-year-olds to learn to read.

What is surprising is that the arguments which raged back and forth were all about methods of teaching reading whereas what was completely absent was any concern about the need for a deeper understanding of what was involved in the process of reading itself. Confronted with public concern about levels of literacy the solution most frequently adopted was to break reading down into more and more subskills with apparatus, aids and kits, exercises and workbooks to instil them.

But the Sentence Method had successfully demonstrated that many children, with skilled and imaginative teaching, could learn by reading for meaning. Phonic methods were often introduced only when children had failed to learn by this approach. However, a closer examination of what, in fact, skilled teachers had been doing all along showed that many of the phonic skills had been introduced incidentally, as the need arose, and that this was most commonly done when children were being taught to write and spell. Similarly, the advocates of a phonic approach could not avoid teaching reading for meaning and introduced this vital component in the written exercises and sentence completion tasks devised to reinforce and monitor the pupils' phonic attack skills and their comprehension of what they had read. In practice, apart from the extremists in both camps, successful teaching of reading combined the best of both approaches. But with no unifying concept of the process of reading, other than an intuitive one, many teachers and parents remained, and often still remain, uncertain and insecure. When the approaches and their methods work everything is fine, but when they fail, whether with individual children or with large groups of socially deprived children, insecurity and an inadequate understanding of the reading process may well result in defensiveness.

The language experience model

If the sentence reading-for-meaning model is in complete contrast to the phonic subskills model, then the language experience model is refreshingly the antithesis of them both.

The language experience model looks like this:

THOUGHT → ORAL LANGUAGE → WRITTEN LANGUAGE → READING

In the classroom or home the sequence began most commonly with a child painting or drawing a picture. Asked about the picture the child might respond by saying, "Mum is digging the garden" or "Dad is feeding the baby". Whatever the child said was written down and read back. "There, now you can trace what you said about your pictures," the child was told. The child, having traced the print, was then asked to read what he had written. Gradually, tracing was replaced by copying what the adult had written. As the children became more proficient in writing and knowledge of the letters, their sounds and graphemic–phonemic patterns, a dictionary might well be built up in which the words were entered. Soon the children would be able to say what they wanted to write down and to write it with very little help, save with new words, from parent or teacher. The language experience model was frequently characterized by words to the effect that, "I know what I mean when I read what I wrote because I knew what I meant when I wrote it". The development of this encoding of thought and language in print was usually the introduction of reading books, but in some schools this was preceded by "language exchange". Children began reading what other children in the class, and then in other classes, had written.

Although, initially, the method suffered from being over-sold as a cure-all in the States, by 1970 it had demonstrated its effectiveness, been widely adopted in schools on both sides of the Atlantic, had received support from the evaluation of its effectiveness by some researchers and had a coherent rationale. Of course, many teachers and parents had been using this approach successfully for decades when they taught children to write their own names, put captions on their pictures and first tell and then write down their "news". But for the first time a model had been introduced which goes back to the beginnings of man's history, to the time when a blaze on a tree or knots in strips of leather served as an *aide memoire*. Man made a mark and remembered what it meant. The later codification of marks into writing systems was but an extension of the concept that the main use of language is to communicate meaning. By helping children to express their thoughts in language and to record them in print there was no gap between print and meaning. What Vygotsky had identified as "the tremendous lag between the school child's oral and written language" and "the abstract quality of written language that is the main stumbling block" had been removed.

One of the difficulties experienced by some dyslexic children is in decoding print from abstract language. But given the task of encoding a short message using a substitution code, such as A = 1, B = 2, C = 3, etc., they have no difficulty. It is always easier to encode a known message than to decode an unknown message. Parents and teachers who help children to write down what they say, whether or not they are aware of the language experience approach, are not only introducing them to reading for meaning, but also introducing left-to-right sequencing, the components of graphemic–phonemic encoding, the use of capital letters, spaces between words and punctuation, and are "imprinting them with print".

A significant contribution to this approach was made by Sylvia Ashton-Warner, in New Zealand, who encouraged Maori children to tell her their own special word, which was often a word like "kiss" or "ghost", for example. Each child was then given a card on which this special word had been written. By beginning with a word of great importance to the child, Sylvia Ashton-Warner established from the outset that reading and writing were valuable individual activities. The language experience approach is also included as a story-writing activity in the Reading Recovery Programme developed in Auckland, New Zealand.

In England "The Breakthrough to Literacy" Schools Council Project, attempted to simplify the process of the language experience model by providing children with printed cards of selected words which they arranged in sentences of their own devising in a sentence-track. As a "ready-made" this has proved popular and successful particularly with linguistically deprived children and their teachers. Many teachers add to the stock of word-cards by adding words which the children have used orally. However, by using printed word-cards, although this saves teachers' time and effort, much of the impact of the original approach is lost and children do not have the same motivation to develop writing and spelling skills by tracing, copying and writing what has been written especially for them.

The language experience model is the first coherent and comprehensive model of the reading process to emerge. It recreates for the child the complete process of going from thought to speech, thence to encoding in print, and from that print to reading. Objections to the approach are usually concerned with the time-consuming nature of the tasks required of teachers and with the initial limitations of vocabulary and sentence structure imposed by the children. These very limitations of vocabulary and sentence structures are, or course, the great advantage of the approach as they ensure that writing and reading begin at "where the child is" and not at where someone remote from him thinks he should be. It is an excellent model for parents and for teachers working with small groups of children. It is also a vital component of any reading programme. When used by skilled teachers the model is so powerful that the disadvantages are readily overcome and children are able to progress rapidly in reading, writing and spelling. Fortunately, some teachers have always been able to overcome the disadvantage, from which they nearly all suffer, of managing and teaching dozens of children, or what Groucho Marx called society's propensity for "putting ages in cages". Most parents do not have this problem.

Psycholinguistic models

Developments in psycholinguistics over recent decades began to impinge upon the teaching of reading in the 1960s. Psycholinguistics is the study of variations in linguistic behaviour in relation to such psychological factors as memory, attention and perception. In looking at the problems involved in understanding the process of reading, psycholinguistics frequently incorporates concepts from information theory and systems analysis. For the first time since Huey's classic study of reading in 1908, serious attention was given to examining the process of reading as a totality and in depth.

The superficiality of much of the research into and argument about phonics and look-and-say, as if separately or mixed together they were an adequate model or method of reading, contrasts with the detailed analysis to which the process was now subjected. Psycholinguistics distinguishes between the surface structures of spoken and printed language and the deep structure or meaning of language, to which we have already referred. Research has investigated the perceptual aspects of scanning print and the role of memory and psycholinguistics has attempted to explain how these processes contribute to our ability to gain understanding from print. One of the most influential researchers, Goodman, in America, has described reading as a psycholinguistic guessing game in which the various strategies of the reader contribute to the progressive reduction of uncertainty as "the reader strives to *reconstruct*" the meaning of the author. "Reading for meaning" is not seen as a single, self-sufficient ability depending on word recognition, as in the sentence method. Instead, the analysis includes: scanning for the most meaningful cues, which sometimes may be graphemes (the capital letters of names, say), sometimes may be phonemes (to build a "new" word), or morphemes (syllables like "dys-", "un-", "-ology", or "-ness" the meaningful bits of words); anticipation; Short Term and Long Term Memory, and their interaction. In considering Goodman's analysis it is useful to reflect upon the different strategies we use when responding to a single word, such as "Stop!" on a road sign, to a less familiar sentence such as "Eins within a space and a wearywide space it wast ere wohned a Mookse", or to the apparently simple sentence, "To be or not to be, that is the question". In response to "Stop!" we respond as by a reflex action: the word, once perceived, enters Sensory or Short Term Memory and we react without recourse to further cues or thought. James Joyce's sentence requires that we recognize, by whatever route available to us, perhaps the recognition of the German words or of the rhythm of the sentence, the familiar pattern he has orchestrated of "Once upon a time there lived a Mookse". Here Short Term Memory must help us through to the end of the sentence and Long Term Memory must be tapped, but we will also be using phonemic and morphemic cues as well as contextual ones if we are reading it for the first time. Hamlet's sentence, well within the competence of many beginning readers, demands that, to understand it, we integrate it with all that we have accumulated in Long Term Memory about Hamlet's possible reasons for making such a statement and hold it there while we read on to get further amplification of its meaning. We will need long reflection, perhaps, before we decide whether or not he is contemplating suicide or the murder of his uncle.

Reading is thus seen as an active, participatory process. Reconstructing the meaning of the author requires that we use a variety of strategies and cues to reduce uncertainty and gain meaning. For us to persist in the process we must receive continuous confirmation that our guesses have been right. If this does not happen, we become confused, the rate of reading slows and the experienced reader may have to go back and re-read, reach for the dictionary — or find an easier book. Motivation in reading, the maintenance of attention and our involvement in the process as active participants, is another aspect which has concerned psycho-linguists. We must find the process self-rewarding: it must give us the information we want, the pleasure or vicarious experience we need. Without this feed-back, attention wanders and meaning is lost.

The early contributions of psycholinguistics have been amplified by our understanding of the perceptual processes involved. This has shown that it is only what goes on "behind the eyes", rather than "before the eyes", which makes it possible for competent readers to read at about 300 words per minute. In a single glance the brain can only process four or five letters a second. If reading was dependent solely upon our ability to recognize and process indi-vidual letters we would be able to read at only about 60 words a minute. When that is the case, as with beginning readers plodding through print and building up sounds to make words, however, the rate of reading is so slow that memory cannot sustain the load of information and meaning is lost. Little wonder that, having reached the end of the sentence, the children may be unable to say what they have read. Learning to read efficiently involves learning to perceive the most significant cues of print as economically as possible. We look for the most significant characteristics of the most significant letters, look for the most meaningful and signifi-cant chunks of letters in syllables and words, and look for whole phrases and sentences in one glance. Because we can anticipate from these minimal cues, we are able to read quickly, hold large chunks of information in memory and access the meaning of what we have read.

We are helped in this process by our awareness of language, of the way in which words follow one another, of how language expresses thought. We anticipate what the text is about and are cognitively aware of how to scan print for meaning. Downing calls this the "literacy acquisition process". Awareness of language or "cognitive clarity" is a prerequisite for reading. Past and present experience of spoken and written language, of how it is structured, again enables us to anticipate. Clearly a sentence beginning "Although. . ." prepares us to anticipate a different kind of sen-tence from one beginning "When. . .". Downing also points out that not only is cognitive awareness or clarity essential but that, in learning to read, factors extraneous to the act of reading, have a bearing upon how clearly the child understands what is involved in reading. The child's response to teachers, to schooling, to the expectations of parents, teachers and peers, the motivation these may or may not provide, and past success or failure, are all factors which have bearing upon how the child approaches reading.

Lunzer and Roberts relate the contributions of psycholinguistics to the teaching of reading. Following Goodman, they conceptualize reading as "a hierarchical process of uncertainty reduction in which the key level is the identification of words". The primary cues to meaning are the visual graphemic–phonemic elements, the surface structure of print which we process as a perceptual-motor activity. These processing skills, they argue, can and should be largely taught "independently of the reading of text". In other words, for instance, we may teach letter shapes, their names and sounds, in teaching writing or in such games as "I Spy".

But, when we come to teach reading, children should first be encouraged to look for meaning and for contextual cues. With beginning readers, of course, these contextual cues may be pictures, the story they already know or the names of the characters. Only when these do not reduce uncertainty are the various strategies for recognizing words, syllables, letter groups or clusters, brought into play to process unfamiliar words. Thus a child being helped with a "new" word, say, "caravan" or trying to decode "lieutenant" clearly needs a repertoire of strategies. In the case of "lieutenant" relating the end of the word to the contextual cue that the man is a soldier will be a more successful strategy than waiting until teacher reaches Phonic Unscrambling Rule 179 "ieut" = "eft" (Eng) or "oot" (Am)!

Much of the work we have been surveying in this section has been given wide currency by Frank Smith. He recognizes that while the major contribution of psycholinguistics has been a deeper understanding of the process, this does not mean that there is "a psycholinguistic method of teaching reading". He suggests that the good intuitive teacher, who may well be a parent, "who responds to what the child is trying to do" and who interacts with the child as the situation demands at the time, is more effective than one who follows a "method". As we still do not understand the complexities of the ways in which we learn to read, we can only determine that different children learn to read in different ways at different times. In helping them the good intuitive teacher, who has "a feel for what is really going on", will be sensitive to the children's unspoken intellectual demands and encourage and respond to their hypothesis testing. In doing so, we may find that, "Yesterday's methods might even work a little better if we get some insight into what really made them effective".

It is in this context of the importance of helping children to go from the surface structure of print to the deep structure of meaning that we should read Frank Smith's (1973) "12 Easy Ways to make Learning to Read Difficult". As this is often seen as begging the question, "How do you make learning to read easy?" we have attempted an answer.

Figure 1   Twelve easy ways to make learning to read difficult

1. Aim for early mastery of the rules of reading.
2. Ensure that phonic skills are learned and used.
3. Teach letters or words one at a time, making sure each new letter or word is learned before moving on.
4. Make word-perfect reading the prime objective.
5. Discourage guessing; be sure children read carefully.
6. Encourage the avoidance of errors.
7. Interrupt to correct errors.
8. Detect and correct inappropriate eye movements.
9. Identify and give special attention to problem readers as soon as possible.
10. Make sure children understand the importance of reading and the seriousness of falling behind.
11. Take the opportunity during reading instruction to improve spelling and written expression, and also insist on the best possible spoken English.
12. If the method you are using is unsatisfactory, try another. Always be alert for new materials and techniques.

From F. Smith (1973) *Psycholinguistics & Reading*, New York: Holt, Rinehart & Winston.

Figure 2   Twelve easy ways of making learning to read easy

1. Regularly read aloud to the child books that will get the child book-hooked — motivated to learn to read.
2. Encourage the child to follow your finger as it moves along the line of print as you read to develop left–right scanning.
3. Talk together about what you have read to develop understanding, use of the language of print and attentive listening.
4. Get the child to read along with you in unison so that supported reading helps the child to get print-borne. This is paired reading.
5. Play oral word games, such as I Spy, Grandmother's Cat, charades, etc., to develop language consciousness or awareness.
6. Teach the child to write his or her name, family names, names of favourite toys or foods, and later sentences the child has said. If necessary, begin by tracing and copying. The objective is that reading, writing and spelling develop hand in hand as encoding–decoding activities.
7. Build up a repertoire of rhymes and jingles, songs and jokes, which are enjoyed and learned by heart by the child, to develop memory and sequencing skills and a sense of fun in the language game.
8. Write out the rhymes, jingles, etc., and encourage the child to use them as prompts when reading them aloud.
9. Once reading along or paired reading is established, encourage the child to guess what comes next when you pause. This will start to get the child print-borne.
10. Use the books you are reading together to play "Hunt the Word that says . . ./begins with . . ./ends with . . .", to develop selective attention to the characteristics of print and its patterns.
11. Once the child is print-borne, only ask the child to read alone sentences or passages you have first read together and which, you are confident, can be read successfully. This is prepared reading.
12. Make it fun! Praise attention, effort and correct responses. If the child is uncertain give the correct response before anxiety develops. A little and often is better than a lot rarely.

The art of using these ways of making reading easy lies in adapting them to the maturity and interests of the child in a way which respects the child's integrity. In determining where to begin, it is essential to go so far back that the child is confident and secure and able to enjoy success. Make it as easy and as much fun as learning to ride a bike.

The present state of the art provides us with a broad conceptual framework of the process of reading. It is now necessary to develop a model which embraces this, and which attempts both to embody factors which have been neglected and to provide a sufficiently powerful instrument for the teaching of reading. A global or holistic approach to reading must encompass all that we know and which we may only yet dimly perceive of the nature of the process, and all that we know of how children may be helped to learn.

A Holistic model of reading

Reading is more than the sum of its parts. As we have seen, the process is itself a part of language and in reading is encoded the complexity, diversity and richness of thought, language and our culture. *The process of reading does not engage just the eye but our whole personality which, by reading, may be enhanced. To read we must be aware of language, and by reading we are made more aware of language. By participating through our understanding and imagination in reading we may gain in both understanding and in imagination. To conceptualize reading as anything less than this is to demean both it and ourselves.*

Although print is not speech our brains process both and they share, in part, common memories and common neural networks. Even as we read swiftly and silently, microelectrodes can detect suppressed neural activity in our speech organs. Unsure of how to spell a word we write it down quickly in the hope that our hand will show us. Reading is not the same as writing but they are both automatized skills which share the same deep structure of meaning.

A holistic model of reading relates thought and language to speech and to writing. Whereas in the models we have been discussing the subskills of decoding print are either acquired during the experience of reading or are learned independently, many of these subskills may be learned by writing, by encoding language in print. A holistic model embraces a language experience approach and a subskills approach as but different sides of the same coin. The hand and eye which follow the line of print during reading learn the same and other skills during writing. Thus thought and language, reading and writing, develop hand in hand. The reduction of uncertainty of meaning when we read is matched

Figure 3   Holistic model of reading

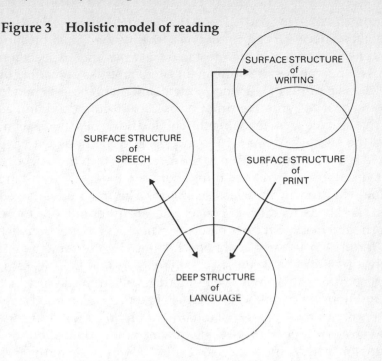

The model shows the relationships between the surface structures of speech writing and print to meaning. Unlike Frank Smith, we show the overlap between the surface structures of writing and of print but, like him, we show the difference between decoding and encoding.

by the certainty of meaning when we write. In reading, the surface structure of print is fixed and is certain but about its meaning we may be uncertain. In writing the endcoding is uncertain but the meaning is certain (Fig. 3).

Reading is, like writing, an individual and solitary act. No one can read for us, they can only read to us; no one can write for us, they can only write at our dictation or instruction. The intervention of another person may impose upon the text a meaning or significance we would not make. Another person may inhibit our thoughts and their flow if that person is not the audience we address in writing. Learning to read is an individual act, too, and the best way and only way to learn is individually with someone to facilitate the process and to prepare our way and guide us towards the goal. No one can learn for us. To learn we must be motivated and the only satisfactory motivation for learning to read is the motivation to learn to read. Given this motivation, and the cognitive abilities necessary in the learner, the teacher must be supportive, encouraging, and manifest to the learner high expectation of success. This can best be done in the ongoing tasks of reading or writing. If, as parents or teachers, we embark on helping a child to learn to read or to write we must be as close to the child and as supportive as if we were teaching the child to ride a bike or to swim. Perhaps the success of any of the models and methods we have discussed is in direct proportion to the extent to which the teachers' skills are used to ensure close contact between themselves and the individual children in the class or group. The most advantaged children, so far as reading is concerned, are undoubtedly those who learned to read with their parents or members of their families before or during the early years of schooling. By the same token, the high correlation between successful readers and large classes, which is so often cited, may well in part result from the fact that these conditions demanded that teachers had to develop good class expectations of literacy, high standards of organization and control, and group methods of working in which individual attention, as Professor M. Vernon urges, could be given. Southgate's research, to which we referred earlier, is relevant here.

Reading and the curriculum

A holistic approach must, therefore, recognize that individual children learn in individual ways and provide for a variety of approaches. This is not to advocate eclecticism but to demand clarity about the variety of strategies by which children may find meaning in print and by which they may learn and be helped to learn. This, in schools, is a part of the curricular process in which aims and objectives are clearly planned to achieve expected and unexpected outcomes with flexibility and sensitivity. If this is to be done then the Physical, Intellectual, Emotional, Cultural, Educational and Social abilities and needs of each child must be considered before we can devise the Short-term, Realizable and Relevant, INteresting Goals, what we have called the PIECES OF STRING, which will achieve the objective of the enjoyment and use of reading and our aims of literacy as a language for life.

Two aspects of the meaning of print have not been adequately stressed but are essential at all levels with the exception, possibly, of the beginning reader for whom they are provided by the parent or teacher. First, in reading we are enabled to go beyond the information given. What we gain in meaning is in direct proportion to the language and thought, ideas and imagination, knowledge and intellectual skills, we bring to the act. But, by reading, we may extend or develop these faculties and also make inferences or judgments which were not in the text or in the author's mind. The second aspect of the search for meaning is that the result of the search should be rewarding. Whether we are looking in our diaries for a date, reading Plato's *Republic*, a novel or a micro manual, we need the continuous feed-back of information or pleasure. These aspects of reading make the activity a self-rewarding one. Without them the search becomes tedious and although the words flash by our eyes they do not impinge upon us beyond the stage of sensory or Primary Memory. With experience we will use selective attention and "skip-read". But the child in the early stages of reading who is fed only the pabulum of primers or basal readers which fail to engage the interest or imagination will be denied the motivation to go on reading and seek the far richer diet of comics or derring-do. The child may write reading off and switch the TV on.

A holistic instructional model

In a holistic model of reading the process is defined as follows:

> Reading is the automatised, self-rewarding, cultural activity of par-
> ticipating in the retrieval of thought and language encoded in alpha-
> betic symbols by left to right lateral scanning so that, when decoded
> and synthesised into words, the words in their contexts give access
> to meaning.

In order to develop an instructional model of reading we must go beyond the definition. Clearly, there can be no one method of instruction but a selection of a variety of means to achieve the ends. The child must above all be familiar with the process, value it highly and be strongly motivated to acquire the skill. In the acquisition of the skill the learner must be supported and assured of success by success. Familiarity with the decoding of print must entail the development of a variety of individual strategies for informed guessing at meaning. Insight into decoding and into the process of reading must be given by helping the child to encode thought and language in writing: "What I say I can write, and what I wrote I can read" as in the language experience model. In the development of the skill the close interaction of the teacher must facilitate the learner's progression from passive to active reading, from competence to achievement, and from achievement to mastery. At all levels and in all activities, including writing and spelling, adequate practice must contribute to the development of efficient memorization and automatization. Throughout instruction the learner's self-esteem must be enhanced by the knowledge of the parent's or teacher's high expectation and of the results of the effort being made. Increasingly, as the skill develops, the learner must be motivated by the self-improving and self-rewarding nature of reading. At all times, therefore, regard must be given to what is going on within the learner.

In Fig. 4 we indicate the main components of the complex of perceptuo-motor, cognitive, memory, processing and motivating activities within the learner. Outside the black-box are all the environmental factors of home, school, peer groups, the media and our culture. Within the box are also the developmental, emotional, attitudinal, intellectual and autonomic factors which may affect or impinge upon the learner. The circles represent the perceptuo-motor activities involved in hearing and speaking language and in reading and writing print. They operate at the surface level of consciousness when stimulated either externally or when set in action as the result of intrinsic motivation. For the system to work, the individual must, in other words, be aroused. This alone ensures that attention is focused upon the activities and that learning can take place. When attention is focused upon a specific activity, neural processes in turn activate memory, thereby giving access to the deep structure of thought and language and to the coding and decoding skills. Within memory, too, is stored experience of all the perceptuo-motor activities and, when active, the experience of one sense or modality can call upon experience stored in the other senses. Thus, in speaking we use auditory or visual information to which we are attending and to which we have attended. Learning tasks must facilitate this inter-sensory or cross-modal interaction and integration. However, this must be done in

Figure 4 Holistic model of the process of reading, writing and spelling

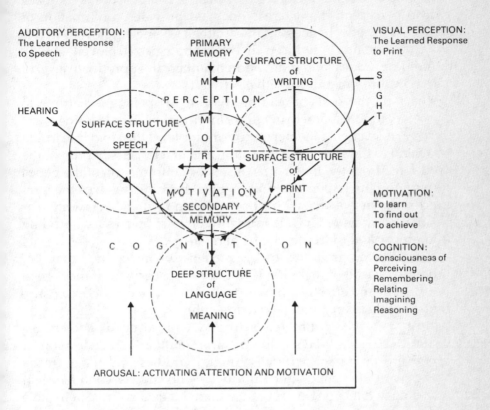

By imposing the model of the levels of language upon a model of the complex of perceptuo-motor, cognitive, memory and processing systems and of arousal and motivational activities involved in reading, we derive the Holistic Model. Outside the black box and immediate perception are all the environmental factors of home, the media, culture, peer groups, etc.; and within it are also the developmental, emotional, autonomic, attitudinal and intellectual, etc. factors involved.

Interacting with the learner, responding to what the child is trying to do, assumes both adequate internal motivation and the ability to form hypotheses, and to test them, on the part of the learner. By whatever path we facilitate learning to read, the child must be enabled to find meaning in the deep structure of language.

such a way as to avoid conflict of attention or interference of one sense of modality with another, as in the case of attempting to read and to watch television or of reading aloud with expression while scanning a text the meaning of which is still obscure. Feed-back to the perceptuo-motor areas engaged provides confirmation or denial of the effectiveness of the strategies being employed. In this way uncertainty is reduced or other strategies deployed. At the same time arousal and motivation maintain an appropriate level of perceptuo-motor and cognitive activity.

Learning the skills of reading, writing or spelling is learning to perceive, to access and to integrate information. This learning is at a variety of levels. At the perceptuo-motor level the child is learning to attend to the visual and meaningful characteristics of print or the feed-back from the finger-tips of sensory information of the pencil moving on the paper. At another level, learning involves the integration of what is seen with what is said and with what is written or heard. At a deeper level, learning involves strategies for encoding in memory and for retrieving from memory.

Planning programmes of instruction, whatever they may be, must involve all of these kinds and levels of learning. If they are to be efficient and effective, however, they must be planned to ensure that all of them are optimized to meet the diversity of children. The parent who talks with, reads to and with, a child, encourages writing activities, plays I Spy or Grandmother's Cat, develops a repertoire of nursery rhymes, jingles, riddles and jokes, reads along with the child, and gradually encourages confidence in guessing what word or sentence comes next, is in the enviable position of getting the child book-borne in the happiest of circumstances. Teachers must plan for more constrained circumstances.

MODES of Reading

Some years ago, when we were designing a computer-assisted learning project for retarded readers, we had to address ourselves to this problem of meeting the needs of a diversity of children who, we knew, would learn by a diversity of strategies. To meet their needs and to allow them to learn by a variety of modes we planned activities in a gentle gradient of difficulty in five areas. For convenience, we called the areas Modes as this suggested to teachers that they were but different paths to the same objective and also indicated that different senses or modalities were involved.

Mode **M**   The Main Mode to Meaning in which more able readers initially, and all children eventually, learn to read by reading.

Mode **O**   The Orthographic and Calligraphic Mode in which children learn the patterns of writing and spelling and gain cues to the encoding and decoding of print.

Mode **D**   The Dialogue Mode in which the children's self-concept, task orientation to reading, arousal of interest and knowledge of teacher expectation is developed.

Mode **E**   The Language Experience Mode in which children encode language in writing.

Mode **S**   The Subskills Mode to reading in which the children's auditory and visual discrimination, memory, scanning, decoding and retrieval skills are developed to assist the process of uncertainty reduction by using cues in their search for meaning.

The games and activities in each mode all converged upon reading for meaning and the programme allowed for various speeds of learning and progress. The details of the system need not concern us here, but its salient features, we suggest, are essential components of any programme designed to meet the needs of children who are experiencing difficulties in learning to read. These salient features, we recognize, of course, are embodied in the practice, in some form or another, of all effective teachers of reading who are not wedded to a particular method or box of tricks.

When difficulties arise for children in learning to read, in the vast majority of cases this is due to the fact that they have been given opportunities to learn only in a narrow and often inadequate and inappropriate range of experiences. Often, when this is realized, all that happens is that efforts are redoubled to teach the skill or subskill in which children are deficient and have experienced failure. This is like rubbing a puppy's nose in his dirt: we rub their noses in print.

In the case of many dyslexic pupils attempts to help them frequently emphasize decoding phonemes without first helping them to learn to encode their own language in writing. Again, the persistence of the difficulties these children have with spelling, after they have learned to read, may well be a product both of the years of reading experience they have missed and of an over-concentration on reading in isolation from those activities of writing and spelling which contribute to it and are properly a part of the process and of the instructional model derived from it.

Reading is an acquired and a complex skill. Each child masters it in a way that is individual and unique. When children fail to learn to read it is more reasonable to assume that we have failed to find a way of helping them which is appropriate to their needs than to assume that the fault lies within the children. For this reason, when we turn to examine the research into dyslexia and children's reading difficulties, our assessment of that research must be informed by judgments about how comprehensively and insight-fully the researchers themselves have conceptualized the process of reading. The difficulties most commonly ascribed to dyslexic pupils and to children described as having "specific retardation in reading" are largely concerned with problems with the processing of the surface structure of print. Some researchers, however, stress the language processing difficulties that some of these children have. Such difficulties are with the deep structure of thought and language. In Fig. 5 we itemize these difficulties and indicate their independence. We also suggest how these difficulties relate to the problems many beginning readers have in learning to read, and to the difficulties experienced by linguistically deprived pupils. Without an adequate and comprehensive understanding of those aspects of the process of reading at present accessible to us there is a real danger that we may fail to understand the nature or the significance of these children's difficulties and needs.

Figure 5   Check-list — why they can't read
Difficulties commonly identified in dyslexic and reading retarded children

SURFACE STRUCTURE FACTORS

Difficulties with left–right directionality of print.
Difficulties with spatial orientation of print (reversals).
Abnormal eye-movements when scanning print.
Slow response to visually presented material.
Poor short-term memory for sequences.
Lack of dominance of visual over auditory stimuli.
Poor cross-referencing of visual and auditory information.
Difficulties in synthesizing sounds to words.
Attentional difficulties.
Poor whole word recognition.
Poor pattern recognition of print.
Persistent spelling difficulties.

DEEP STRUCTURE FACTORS

Poor ability to name objects.
Poor ability to categorize objects.
Poor long-term memory for complex information.
Inadequate knowledge of word meanings and of morphemes.
Inadequate knowledge of the syntax or structure of language.
Lack of verbal fluency.
Difficulties in the automatization of reading.

Any one or more of the difficulties with Surface Structure Factors may prevent a child from gaining meaning from print. If all Surface Structure Factors are processed satisfactorily and the difficulties exist in Deep Structure Factors the child will read without adequate understanding and be confused.

Difficulties with Surface Structure Factors are common in beginning readers and in children who have received inadequate instruction. Deep Structure Factors are those with which linguistically deprived children have difficulty.

Difficulties with both Surface and Deep Structure Factors are susceptible to correction by appropriate instruction and incentives.

CHAPTER 4

Dyslexia and Research

"There is no scientific study more vital to man than the
study of his own brain. Our entire view of the universe
depends on it."   F.H.C. Crick

An overview

Dyslexia is a controversial, fascinating and perplexing subject
because it raises fundamental questions about the nature of man as
a speech-using animal, and about the brain of which we know so
little. Unfortunately, however, even a selective bibliography of the
research into dyslexia would occupy the whole of this book and any
adequate treatment of one single aspect of that research would
require more than this chapter. Moreover, that treatment would
have to assume that the reader already understood something of
the disciplines involved and the principles of research design. All
that we can attempt to do is to provide an overview of the main
lines of enquiry and its problems and then to examine some of the
questions often asked by parents and professionals who have not
had opportunity to explore the subject in depth. The standpoint
from which we view the problem is that dyslexic children and
children with severe reading difficulties, no matter what the causes
and nature of their disabilities, are like the millions of illiterate and
semiliterate children in the world: they have not had adequate and
appropriate incentives and opportunities to learn to read. We consider this perspective relevant and timely. *Vast and complex though*

68

the literature may be, what is of paramount importance is that we should identify the special educational needs of these children and be better equipped to meet them.

No research literature could be more difficult to review than that concerned with dyslexia. The subject is not only controversial, it is diffuse and involves many disciplines from biochemistry to zoology, and it is bedevilled by the fact that specific developmental dyslexia is variously defined and there is little agreement about either its nature or its characteristics. There is no guarantee that research literature with dyslexia in the title is concerned with the same concept of the problem as that accepted by other investigators. Nor can it be assumed that the children described by one investigator are similar to those described by another. Furthermore, because the term dyslexia is unacceptable to many reputable researchers, their work in studying reading and learning difficulties cannot be ignored but must be given careful examination. But the biggest difficulty of all is that the research, from no matter what point it may start, inevitably leads into areas in which there are few certainties and in which speculation is rife. This is no reflection upon the work of the dedicated researchers, who have difficulties enough with the often inadequate test instruments and techniques at their disposal, but a reflection upon how little is known and understood about the brain and its processes.

The reading brain

Since acquired dyslexia, or alexia, was first identified over one hundred years ago it has been the subject of almost continuous and detailed investigation. This research has contributed to our understanding of how our brains process language. Today we have a fairly detailed, but by no means complete, knowledge of the main areas of the brain involved in speech, in the understanding of spoken language, in reading and in writing. We know that in the majority of, but not all, people, speech and language processes are largely performed in the left half or hemisphere of the brain. In man the left hemisphere is more developed, both in function and in size, than the right hemisphere. At its most simplistic, we may say that Broca's area is concerned with speech and the coding of language into its spoken form; Wernicke's area is involved in processing

language that has been received through the ears; and an area
called the angular gyrus, in association with the other two areas, is
concerned with written forms of language, (Fig. 6). Much of this
knowledge has been gained by the investigation of patients suffering from injuries to the brain. The maimed of two world wars,
victims of accidents, strokes and tumours, have all contributed to
the detailed mapping of the discrete areas of the brain involved in
the various language and other processes of the brain. More
importantly, they have illuminated the ways in which the different
processes interact with one another.

However, it is axiomatic in neurology that a damaged brain
provides only a damaged model of normal functioning. We can no
more assume, on the evidence of a lesion to the brain and an effect
upon the patient's peformance, that there is a direct relationship
between them, than we can assume that, when a car suddenly
stops and the ignition light comes on that it is the ignition light

Figure 6   The brain

Diagram of the main areas involved in speaking, writing, listening to and
reading language

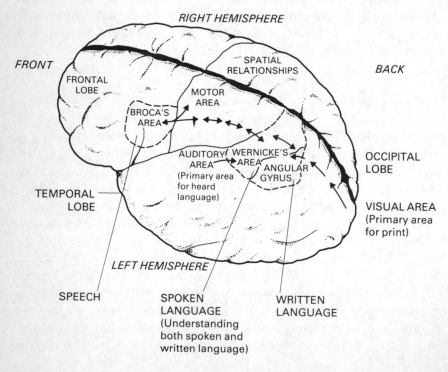

which powers the car. Studies of brain-damaged patients have had to be related to findings from electrical and chemical stimulation of the brain, from monitoring the brain's activity by means of micro-electrodes, and from studies of the wave patterns of cerebral activity by means of electroencephalography (EEG). Similarly, our understanding of the brain has been informed by investigations into the biochemistry of neural transmission, by psychiatry and psychology. It is important to stress this because much of the literature concerned with reading difficulties in children has tended to assume that these difficulties could be directly compared with pathological conditions in adult patients who had suffered cerebral insult. Medical students frequently go through a phase of thinking that they have all the symptoms of which they read in their text-books and, indeed, some of them may have some of the symptoms. But it is also axiomatic that in scientific investigation one should look first for the simplest feasible explanations rather than the most remote and obscure ones. When the car stops we don't begin by dismantling the gear-box: we first check the tank.

Acquired dyslexia and language disorders

Certainly, in most cases of acquired dyslexia or alexia in adults, and in cases of patients with other language difficulties resulting from cerebral lesions, neurology enables us to understand a great deal about the cerebral processes affected. They can explain why a lesion in the area of the angular gyrus affects the ability to read; they can explain why some patients have difficulty in expressing themselves in speech, expressive aphasia or dysphasia, while others cannot respond to spoken instructions, receptive aphasia. It is now possible to understand why cerebral damage which renders an English-speaking patient unable to read may have much less effect upon Chinese or Japanese patients' reading ability. This detailed knowledge, however, cannot account for the reading or language difficulties of children for whom there is no evidence of cerebral damage. At best it may provide some insights into possible factors involved in their difficulties. Some research into reading problems in children has been concerned to examine whether the children present other manifestations of malfunction or dysfunction which may be attribual to neurological factors.

Handicapped children and reading difficulties

Knowledge of the cerebral processes involved in reading enables us to better understand the difficulties of children handicapped at, during or shortly after birth by asphyxia, cerebral palsy, encephalitis or meningitis. The spastic hemiplegic whose left side and limbs are affected may well have no difficulties with language or with reading. A hemiplegic whose right side and limbs are in spasm *may* have both language and reading difficulties. This is because, as we have seen, the language areas of the brain are usually in the left hemisphere which controls the right side of the body. Children who have suffered damage to both hemispheres may well have both sides of the body affected and have speech and language problems. But even with children about whom there is no doubt that they have suffered considerable damage to their brains and have little control over their limbs, it is wrong to assume that they cannot develop thought and language, reading and, with some form of aid, writing abilities. Studies of the abilities, rather than the disabilities, of these handicapped children, young people and adults, and of the visually, hearing and mentally impaired, have demonstrated the plasticity, adaptability and complexity of cerebral processes. We remember, in this connection, seven-year-old Jake in a Diagnostic Assessment Unit. Jake had a limited repertoire of two-word utterances and very strange noises. In every respect he functioned like a large and violent two-year-old. Observation showed he was never still for longer than 7 seconds. Further observation surprisingly revealed that Jake could read and that he understood what he read. This hitherto unknown fact about Jake, which like everything else about him no one could explain, is the other side of the coin. We don't know why some children cannot read, and we have no adequate explanation of how some children do read.

Work with handicapped children also shows that some of them have reading difficulties which may arise as a result of the effects of their primary handicap as in the case of epileptic attacks. This has been found to be more commonly the case with boys than girls. But account must also be taken of the fact that some handicapped children have reading difficulties which are in no way connected with their primary disability.

Our understanding of reading and language difficulties has also been informed by the important achievements in the education of children with sensory disabilities, the blind and partially sighted and, particularly, the deaf and partially-hearing. Visual defects not only result in children having to master printed language through the sense of touch or by means of aids which enable them to use their residual vision, they also deny the children, wholly or in part, visual information about their world to which language refers. Yet this rarely has any effect upon their language and cognitive development. Deaf and some severely hearing-impaired children, however, have problems in the reception and acquisition of speech and also in developing an understanding of the complexity and nuances of language. Reading can therefore present a difficult hurdle for them to surmount, but, once surmounted, it provides them with access to language. Studies of these children's difficulties and of those who are autistic or mentally impaired, and the exciting work which has been done to develop communication with and for them, have all contributed to our understanding of language processing and of ways in which it may be disrupted and facilitated.

Neurological development and language

Particularly significant for the better understanding of the educational needs of children with reading, writing and spelling difficulties is the knowledge gained about how the brain grows, changes and develops its abilities to process language and its skills. In the early months of life both sides of the brain are involved in language. By about four years, the left hemisphere has taken over specialization in language processing. Most people, including the many who are left-handed, are left-hemisphere dominant, that is, have the main functions for language and cognitive processes localized in the left side of the brain. However, this does not happen in the case of some right-handed or ambidextrous people. Nor is it true for about 50% of left-handed people. Children who have sustained injury to the left side of the brain in infancy may develop the functions in the right hemisphere. The remarkable plasticity of the brain during infancy is still not fully understood.

Some processes involved in reading develop more slowly than

others. In particular, our perception of whether things or symbols are up or down, on the right or left, is not usually fully developed until about nine years of age. Children who are adept at copying circles, squares, crosses and triangles are rarely able to draw a diamond — represented by a square standing on one corner ◇ — until about six. The frequently observed phenomenon of children reversing letters such as "b", "d", "p" and "q", or words such as "on" and "no", is not surprising, therefore. What is surprising is the number of people who never develop adequate spatial orientation, as it is called, yet lead normal lives. They use other cues to learn to read and to find their way about but, if asked to tell us the way, should we stop them in the street, they may well become inarticulate arm-wavers. Their ability to hold down jobs, whether as surgeons or truck drivers, is illustrative of the way the brain can learn to process information which is distorted or incomplete. All that we know about how the brain learns to perceive and interpret the input from our senses supports this view. Experimenters, given lenses to wear that turned the world upside-down, found that their brains soon learned to turn the images the right way up. When the lenses were removed, at first their world appeared upside-down. Gradually, their brains learned to put the world the right way up again.

From the earliest months of life the brain is learning to check one sense against another. The "What is it?" response in babies demonstrates this: a sudden noise and a baby turns its head and looks in the direction from which the noise came. Talk to a baby and its remarkable sensitivity to language has been shown to evoke waves of neural activity which spread through its whole body. Soon babies are practising making the sounds and rhythms of the language they hear around them.

By the age of four it has been said that children not only have a considerable vocabulary but have mastered, given the opportunity to hear and use them, nearly all the syntactical structures — the grammatical conventions — of language. The language they learn is that of their environment.

Certainly by five or six years most children have virtually all the processes established for learning to read if they have not already cracked the code for themselves. Again this skill is gained by associating what they hear with what they see. Clearly, if they have not been exposed to written language in the stories that their parents, older siblings and others read to them, this will not usually happen. As we have seen, being read to does more than teach the brain to attend to letters which stand for sounds: the brain learns to interpret the left to right sequence, to expect meaning from the language which is being decoded and to attend to the patterns of language and of print simultaneously.

In the past it was frequently repeated in the literature that dyslexia was not a learning disability. Certainly, it may not be a general deficiency in learning, but failure to learn to read must of necessity evidence a failure to learn to decode language from print. As in all perceptual activities, the brain has to learn to process the information received.

Models of the brain

Neurology began as speculation and then, from what neurologists call the "splendid seventies" of the last century, began the careful mapping of discrete areas of the brain, which endeavoured to assign each function of the body and its senses to specific locations. It was all very much like the phrenological "bumps" view of the head that it was replacing. The search still goes on and one area, in the right hemisphere, identified a few years ago, is specifically involved in our recognition of faces. Increasingly, however, it became clear that the brain is far more complex than was at first thought. Areas may have a variety of functions, and the basic "building block" of the brain, the neuron, is unlike any other cell in the human body. It is estimated that our brains consist of 10,000,000,000 neurons, each of which is different from the others. One neuron may be connected to up to 10,000 other neurons by synapses. Schwann cells surround the connecting axons of the neurons in a myelin sheath involved in speeding up transmission of impulses from neuron to neuron. The rest of the brain consists of cells, called glia, which support and feed the neurons. The role of the glial cells is still not fully understood. What began as a search for a more or less mechanical system to explain the functions of the brain is now a study of its biochemistry.

In order to conceptualize his limited understanding of the brain, man, the only animal to study its brain, has tried to make models to explain it coherently. From gods and planets, which were thought to control it, to philosophical concepts, vapours, and mechanical systems, we have gone on to electrical circuitry, computers, communication theory and systems analysis. In the conceptualization of genetic transmission crystallography was brought in to help to produce the model of the double helix. It is interesting to speculate what new models will be used to explain the biochemistry of the brain. One suggestion is that we should imagine minute aerosols spraying the areas of the cortex to activate them.

Today, the brain is often considered as having three main functional units, interacting with one another as a system. This dynamic system of interacting processes consists of the following units which are involved in all cerebral activity:

Unit 1   The regulation of our level of arousal or wakefulness;
Unit 2   obtaining, processing and storing information from our senses;
Unit 3   programming, regulating and verifying our mental activity.

Thus, the processes we have already described which are involved in language and in reading may, at first glance, be assigned to Unit 2 — obtaining, processing and storing information received through eye and ear. But obviously Unit 1 is also involved: we must attend to and be interested in what we are doing; and we do sometimes fall asleep when reading! Unit 3 is also involved: what we read must be checked against what we know and against what we have read; have we missed the author's meaning or ignored a vital clue to the murderer? Reading cannot be seen as a separate and distinct activity but, like all other mental activity, a part of the total system. Hence the complexity of our holistic model of reading.

Parents and teachers can do little to examine what is going on in their children's angular gyrus, but they can make sure they are comfortable, confident, interested, aroused and alert. They may realize that telling a five-year old her "b" is the wrong way round will not, in itself, correct the error. Instead, they will make a letter "b" and, as they do so, say something like "Here's the straight bat and here's the ball at its feet! Now you make a "b" — first the bat . . ." Arousal and selective attention, programming and regulating, are all involved.

Much of the research literature concerned with specific developmental dyslexia and into retardation in reading is concerned, quite properly, with the processing and storing of visual information from print. Levels of arousal, selective attention and curiosity have less frequently been explored. Similarly, the conscious mental involvement of the pupils' brains in the process of learning to read, Unit 3 in our model, has received inadequate attention. Cracking the code of print, as a game, puzzle or problem-solving activity, and getting to the meaning of the message is part of the process, too. Bright-eyed Ian, keen and co-operative, captain of the football team, top in maths, had used his intelligence to fool everyone he could read — and class after class had aided and abetted him. Now, at eleven, his cover had been blown. "Right, Ian," said his teacher, "I can't teach you to read. You'll have to teach yourself. You can't wait to leave school and join the Air Force can you? Well, this will help you — it's the Morse Code. Here are some messages — when you've worked them out, answer them in code!" It was a very long shot but the teacher knew Ian — and he knew the class would help him! Ian learned to read — and to fly.

Survival and development

We also need to ask ourselves what is the purpose of all these millions of neurons organized into systems. The dynamic model given above gives the clue to this, we suggest. At all levels of its functioning, including sleep, the purpose of the brain is to ensure the survival of the organism in its environment. When we were considering the tremendous growth in language-processing in the early years we touched briefly on the contribution of this interaction of the brain with the language environment of the infant's family. A baby has the potential to learn language, any language, but it is the environment which determines whether it learns Urdu or English, Hebrew or Chinese. Similarly, the skills and abilities the brain develops are largely determined by parents, teachers and society. One child watches TV for five hours a day, another must spend the time gathering brushwood or water, and a third spends one hour playing the clarinet, an hour delivering papers, an hour swimming, an hour reading and an hour programming her computer. Experience and instruction lead development. This is vitally true of learning to write, spell or read. The complexity of this environmental interaction is as great as that of the brain and only a little better understood.

For not only is the brain learning from its experience of its environment, which changes and modifies its processing, it is also changing throughout childhood in preparation for the second bio-chemical explosion of adolescence. Now the potential for pro-creation is matched with a potential for responsibility and for social and intellectual creativity. The capacity for learning is now greatly increased and whole new amplifiers of thought — precepts, concepts, principles, algorithms and new languages — and new disciplines become accessible to conscious control. All this, of course, providing the environment provides the right incentives, stimuli, models and instruction. Children who have been inarticulate may become verbose, those who were verbose may become reflective, those who read avidly seek new experiences for which reading may have prepared them vicariously, and some who could not read cannot be persuaded to get their heads out of their books. Helping the older child to learn to read is difficult. Helping adolescent pupils requires enormous skill, insight, empathy and a willingness to learn from and with them. Finding the right incentives and the right books which will not add to their feelings of failure and inadequacy, is often difficult. Removing the carapaces of avoidance techniques they have developed to protect themselves from exposure and instructing them is an art, which, as Pestalozzi described it: "Depends primarily on the relation and harmony between the impressions to be made upon the child and the specific stage which his developing powers have reached at the time". It is a lack of this art of instruction, we suggest, which in part may account for many older pupils' continuing difficulties.

Indeed, there is little neurological or neuropsychological evidence to explain why some children find reading so difficult. This has not been for want of trying. It is for this reason that we adopt the more economic and parsimonious view that it is seldom that constitutional defects within the children prevent them from learning to read but often the methods of instruction employed to help them.

When we turn to the research into specific developmental dyslexia the reason for this suggestion may appear both less extreme and more cogent. The neurological model of internal processing with which much of the research is concerned needs placing within both the larger model of interacting systems or functions and that model's interaction with environmental factors. The assumption that children's difficulties have a medical or a neurological origin is a reasonable one. But it is only an assumption, a hypothesis. It is the method of science to test hypotheses, theories and laws and to find out when they don't work. Scientific method is less concerned with verification of received knowledge, which may make it little better than dogma, than with discovering its limitations and falsifications.

Limits of neurology

Neurology and neuropsychology only provide us with partial knowledge of the brain and its processes. We are only at the frontiers of understanding the chemistry of the neuron. We know much about the attributes of memory but still do not know how memories are laid down, stored and retrieved. Yet without memory and forgetting we would not long survive. The plasticity of the brain, and the ability of some patients to learn to perform functions after the areas of the brain deemed to control them have apparently been completely destroyed, are by no means fully understood. We cannot account for the fact that some people who have lived normal lives have been found, as the result of autopsies, to have had grossly undeveloped or massively damaged brains. The relationship between the right and left hemispheres and, as we shall see, the nature of cerebral dominance, are still largely unexplored and have only been accessible, in part, to examination in the last thirty years. At a less clinical level, it is difficult to reconcile man's creativity with his destructiveness, his compassion with his cruelty.

We should not be surprised or disappointed, therefore, if we still cannot explain fully why and how we learn to read and why some children and adults find it so unconscionably difficult.

Some problems of research design

Attempts to find an explanation of word-blindness, as it was first called, or specific developmental dyslexia in children, have been made by virtually every school of psychology and psychoanalysis. Behaviourist, gestalt, clinical and developmental psychology have all endeavoured to explain the phenomenon. The main thrust of research, however, has been to identify a single factor or cluster of factors which would demonstrate that it was caused by some constitutional or genetic abnormality or malfunction. Unfortunately, all the research has been beset by the difficulty to which we have already referred: the absence of agreement as to definition. This is a frequent criticism but it should be remembered that different children have different difficulties, the same difficulty may well have a variety of constitutional causes and a variety of manifestations, and each kind of difficulty may have many degrees from mild to severe.

Another problem researchers have had to face is that reading difficulties may be caused by a variety of factors. Having hypothesized that the difficulties are specifically restricted to some constitutional factor involved in the children's internal processing, researchers have had to exclude all other possible factors such as visual defects or school absence. Scientific investigation and experimentation in the laboratory, using pure, genetically bred mice and rats, when all factors can be controlled, are difficult enough. In the real world, researchers have the greatest difficulty. The search for "pure" dyslexics, whose difficulties cannot be accounted for by other factors whether internal or external, entails that researchers must adopt a policy of progressively excluding children from their sample populations. These are some of the common factors on which exclusion is often made:

Visual and hearing disabilities.
Physical defects and handicaps.
Mental handicaps.
Neurological damage.
Below average mental ability.
Below average language development.
Speech defects.
Emotional problems.
Behavioural disorders.
Frequent school changes or absences.
Poor health record.

Disturbed home circumstances.

Social deprivation.

Some of these factors are easy to determine, some can be tested with some degree of reliability but others can not. In many cases the tests are inadequate or suspect by other researchers. Familial and social circumstances are, at best, matters of judgment.

One of the unfortunate by-products of this exclusionary research design has been the widespread misconception that dyslexia is only found in children of above average "intelligence" from "good" homes. This is not the fault of the researchers, but it is a misconception that has been perpetuated, not only by the media, in attempts to dramatize the plight of children with reading diffi-culties. The researchers are well aware that many of the children they have excluded may have specific reading difficulties not accounted for by their other defects, disabilities or handicaps. But in their cases the problem of unravelling what is cause and what is effect would be too complex. Having obtained their sample, a long and time-consuming process, researchers invariably find they have very few children and that within these subjects they have a range of different difficulties. Research in this field is frequently criticized for the small number of children studied and for the lack of consistency, or homogeneity, within the groups.

Hypothetical factors

Whether researchers seek to identify children in this way or pro-ceed with case studies which examine in depth children who have come to clinics or hospitals because of their difficulties, they may well seek to pursue a particular line of enquiry. They will make a hypothesis based on some possible explanation to account for the difficulties. These hypotheses about causation derive from what is known about the neurological and psychological processes in-volved in reading or from models of the reading process itself. Much of the research literature is concerned with examining hypotheses that the children's difficulties may be accounted for by one or more of the following:

Poor or disturbed processing of visual information.

Poor or disturbed processing of auditory information.
Poor or disturbed processing between visual and auditory
   processes.
Memory deficits.
Poor sequencing or ordering.
Difficulties with left and right (laterally).
Difficulties with spatial orientation.
Poorly established cerebral dominance.
Genetic factors.
Biochemical "disorders".
Language difficulties.

The problem for the researcher, whatever hypothesis he investigates, is that rarely is there really firm or "hard" evidence
within the particular subject or discipline involved. As we have
seen, nearly all this research is at the frontiers of our knowledge of
the brain. This is the case with one of the most fundamental
questions frequently asked about dyslexia: is it genetic in origin,
does it run in families? This question arises for three reasons:
natural parental interest; the fact that definitions of specific
developmental dyslexia often state that it may be or is usually
genetically determined; because there appears to be evidence that
there is a familial factor involved. This, and similar questions
frequently asked about dyslexia, we will now examine in the light
of the research.

CHAPTER 5

Questions of Research
and Dyslexia

"When a thing ceases to be a subject of controversy, it
ceases to be a subject of interest."   William Hazlitt

Does dyslexia run in families?

Our genetic inheritance is determined when a half set of chromosomes from the male sperm unites with a half set of chromosomes
from the female ovum. Our forty six chromosomes contain the
genes in which deoxyribonucleic acid, DNA, carries the coded
information for the production of the proteins which will control
the development of a unique individual. Ribonucleic acids, RNA,
act as transmitters or messengers, transfer and binding agents, and
ensure that the coded information is transformed, by protein
synthesis, into a new baby. The chance way in which chromosomes from each parent combine, cell division, "mistakes" in the
chromosomes and, very occasionally, mutations, ensure that
children are different from their parents. Similarly, it accounts for
the fact that children of the same parents are different from one
another. The exception, of course, is that of identical twins who are
similar because of division of the fertilized egg at some stage, before
or after implantation. Genetic inheritance, then, is not only about
the transmission of coded information which will ensure that a new
human being is produced, it is also about ensuring that the new
human being is unique in that it combines a new permutation of
the inherited characteristics of both parents. And from the moment

of conception, when our uniqueness is determined, we are subject to environmental influences which modify our development. Genes need an environment in which to grow. In the womb, development may be affected by the mother's health, by her diet and by such factors as drugs she has been prescribed or whether or not she smokes. During birth other events may intervene which may drastically affect development. Thereafter, the best that can be said, in the words of the geneticist Dobzhansky, is that our "genes determine the reactions of the organism to its environment".

Sorting out what is the result of inheritance and what the result of environmental influences is difficult for geneticists because there are so few characteristics which can reliably be studied. Skin and eye-colour, our blood group, hair colour and, within broad limits, our physique are susceptible to study. In the same way, dramatic variations in human characteristics such as albinism, haemophilia and other diseases have been shown to be the result of inheritance. Less dramatic characteristics which have been studied are colour-blindness, attached ear lobes, which fascinated Darwin, baldness in men, the shape of lips and noses and webbed feet. But because a family shares similar environmental influences, a similar diet, the same atmosphere and similar social strains and stresses or advantages, we can rarely assume that characteristics of a less demonstrably specific kind are inherited. It was once thought that pellagra, which causes wasting and mental depression, was inherited because it ran in families. Then it was shown that, in fact, it was a vitamin B niacin deficiency in the diet of poor families. There is no doubt about the evidence that dyslexia runs in families but determining whether or not it is determined by genetic or environmental factors is a highly complex matter.

Research into the hereditability of reading difficulties has followed four main lines of investigation: family histories, the association of reading difficulties with other genetically determined characteristics, similarities of a biochemical nature, and twin studies.

Family histories provide the most persuasive evidence. Unfortunately, this evidence is largely anecdotal. The fact that a parent reports that father or grandmother had similar difficulties only becomes reliable evidence when we can satisfy ourselves about the nature and causation of father's or grandmother's difficulties. Studies of family histories rarely go back for more than two or three generations and rarely provide adequate data. These data are even less convincing when it is remembered that only a few generations ago, during the Second World War, 20% of recruits to the British forces were classified as semi-literate. Go back four or five generations and we find that about 40% of couples signed their names with a cross when they registered their marriages. Family histories of literacy reflect historical influences and it is well to remember that, on both sides of the Atlantic, in Britain and the USA, universal education and mass literacy began only in the latter half of the last century.

There is ample evidence that children's academic achievements are strongly associated with environmental factors such as the size of the family, social class and material circumstances, parents' reading habits and the number of books in the home. Children's reading ability is particularly associated with whether or not mothers and fathers read to their children and with the frequency with which they hear them read. Research undertaken in connection with the Plowden Report, *Children and their Primary Schools* (1967, HMSO), demonstrated that parents' interest in their children's education was the most significant factor in the level of children's academic achievement.

What can be said with certainty is that dyslexia and reading difficulties run in families and that boys, in a ratio of about 4 boys to 1 girl, are most commonly affected. This phenomenon of a sex difference we examine later. But it is impossible to assign responsibility to genetic factors on the grounds of incidence. This is not to deny the possibilities of a genetic link in some cases, but the evidence does underline the importance of familial and social influences. We can't change children's DNA codes but we can change their environments.

The association of reading difficulties with other genetically determined characteristics has, therefore, been pursued with more rigour by researchers. They have, however, had to contend with the problems of the absence of agreed criteria of dyslexia and of finding co-existent genetically determined signs. For instance, handedness — whether we are right-handed, left-handed or ambidextrous — has been investigated as a possible factor associated with reading difficulties. The evidence for an association is inconclusive and some studies have found that left-handed pupils are in no way inferior to right-handed pupils in reading. There is, however, some association between ambidexterity and reading difficulties; but ambidexterity is difficult to determine, especially in young pupils, with certainty. Ambidexterity raises the problem of cerebral dominance which, as we shall see, is also difficult to resolve. There is no certainty, however, that handedness is an inherited characteristic although in some instances it does appear to be.

Family studies in which there is a history of both dyslexia and epilepsy are sometimes cited but are discounted on the ground that the epilepsy, rather than a genetic factor, caused the brain damage which accounted for the reading difficulties. Sibling studies of the brothers and sisters of dyslexic children have found that the siblings are more likely than the siblings of successful readers to have reading problems. This research fails to distinguish adequately between social and hereditary factors. However, a higher incidence of reading difficulties has been found in siblings of handicapped children receiving special education. There is no evidence of dyslexia being associated with inherited chromosomal abnormality such as that which causes Down's syndrome in children, and there is no evidence of which we are aware that identifies a characteristic or characteristics associated with it. It is surprising that this should be the case in a disability which has attracted so much medical and psychological interest and which is so frequently claimed to be inherited. The possibility that dyslexia itself is the one genetically determined characteristic is not excluded, however.

Biochemical similarities of dyslexic children have been identified in a few studies. As DNA carries the genetic code and RNA translates that code into proteins, investigations have been made into the biochemistry of dyslexics' metabolism. These investigations have sought to identify abnormal functioning. There is evidence that some dyslexics had higher thyroxine levels and, in another study, that their processing of enzymes was different from that of able readers. These factors are significant in neural transmission but it has not been shown whether the differences were the cause or the effect of their learning difficulties. Nor has it been established whether or not they are transmitted genetically. This approach to the problem may produce more significant evidence when we have a more detailed knowledge of the brain's biochemistry but at present it is difficult to imagine a pathological metabolic condition which would have no adverse effect upon learning or performance except in learning to read.

Identical twins share a common set of genes and, therefore, are beloved of researchers. This is because, if they are brought up in different environments, it is possible to sort out characteristics which are genetic from those which result from their different circumstances. Unfortunately, identical twins are uncommon, about one pair in 300 births, and identical twins who are dyslexic are even more uncommon. All that has been established so far is that identical twins show the same reading difficulties, whereas dissimilar twins only share reading difficulties in three case out of ten. The evidence that identical twins share the same difficulties in the same or in different environments, however, is not conclusive of genetic inheritance unless one can be sure that they have not suffered from perinatal disturbances to which twins are more likely to have been subject than singletons. And identical twins, unlike dissimilar twins, do not run in families.

Conclusions Therefore, the evidence that dyslexia runs in families justifies the hypothesis that it may be genetically determined. Such evidence as there is at present, however, does not confirm this. The evidence from a small number of twin studies and from biochemical investigations does not justify making generalizations about dyslexics or children with reading difficulties as a group. Even if it is one day possible to account for the fact that dyslexia runs in families, by demonstrating a genetic link, it will still be necessary to account for the reading difficulties of children in families which have no history of such difficulties. But as reading is an acquired skill or characteristic, unless one adopts a Lamarckian view, there can be no genetic explanation of the mechanism by which reading difficulties are inherited. What is most likely to account for the fact that these difficulties run in families is undoubtedly the influence of environment. In this connection, it is well to remember that parental expectation, like teacher expectation, has a highly significant effect upon a child's performance. In other words, expecting Georgina or George to have difficulties in reading because father or Uncle Geoff had them is highly likely to ensure that they will. We should change the environment and our exectations, we suggest. Characteristics of behaviour, such as reading difficulty, are no more likely to be determined genetically than other behaviours such as our habits or the language we speak. At best, it may be that children inherit some predisposition to having difficulties in reading, accounted for by some or all of the factors we shall examine. Until dyslexia in children can be discretely defined and until it can be shown, as clearly as it is with genetically determined deafness or blindness, for instance, that it may be genetic in origin, it is a misuse of the term "genetic" to include it in any definition or description of the difficulties. Deafness is not defined as a genetic handicap just because research has shown that a proportion of cases of deafness, usually put at between 40% and 60%, are genetic in orgin. No useful purpose is served by compounding children's language difficulties by using language so loosely.

Why do more boys than girls have reading difficulties?

The statistical evidence undoubtedly confirms the impression many teachers and parents have that specific developmental dyslexia and reading retardation are more common in boys than in girls. Most studies cite ratios of between 3 and 5 boys to 1 girl. This has suggested to some researchers that dyslexia might be sex-linked genetically, like haemophilia or some forms of colour-blindness. Sex is determined by what are called the X and Y chromosomes, one from each parent. Women have two X chromosomes (XX); men have one X and one Y chromosome (XY). The little Y chromosome has its genes so packed with DNA, coded to ensure that all the primary and secondary characteristics of maleness develop that it is not thought to carry any other information. Sex-linked defects are transmitted on X chromosomes only. If a woman inherits a single defective X chromosome from her father which, say, might cause colour-blindness, her other X chromosome from her mother will ensure that she has normal vision. However, her sons have a fifty–fifty chance of inheriting her defective chromosome: they may get her normal X chromosome or her defective one. Only in the unlikely event of a girl receiving a defective X chromosome from her mother and another defective X chromosome from her colour-blind father will she be colour-blind. In other words, the odds are stacked against the boys in this kind of sex-linked characteristic.

It has been suggested that this association between dyslexia and boys is accounted for by the fact that not only is the ratio of boys to girls what one might expect if the characteristic were sex-linked, but that in one sample of dyslexic boys from families in which dyslexia was said to be present, all the boys had highly developed spatial abilities. This was said to create difficulties for them in their perception of letters in two dimensions only. However, most boys develop spatial abilities earlier than girls and it is difficult to understand how the highly developed spatial abilities of these boys could constitute more than a temporary stumbling block.

Without suggesting that the characteristic is sex-linked, other research has underlined this developmental difference in spatial perception as a factor in boys' reading difficulties. Other developmental differences argue, on the other hand, that boys' difficulties can be attributed to the fact that they develop more slowly than girls and that, in particular, they lag behind girls in their language acquistion and development. Boys have a greater vulnerability than girls to defects acquired perinatally and have more emotional difficulties in childhood. Girls, at least in the early years, tend to be more conforming than boys and respond more readily to women teachers who, of course, preponderate in playgroups, nursery classes and often in schools until children are nine or more years of age. Boys tend to reject female models of behaviour and seek to identify with their fathers and with peer-group models. It has been pointed out, too, that primers or basal readers are often more attractive to girls than to boys. It was, after all, a girl who protested that, "Johnnie is only reading the pictures!" and a boy who responded, "The words are only for the dopes who don't understand the pictures!" Mark Twain identified part of the problem: "Monday morning found Tom Sawyer miserable. Monday morning always found him so, because it began another week's slow suffering in school." And Tom Sawyer could read.

However, despite all these factors, most boys do learn to read and evidence does suggest that, in fact, the reading levels of boys are often found to be higher than those of girls of the same age. That there are more boys with *early* difficulties in reading in part accounts for the fact that there are more boys with persistent difficulties. A compounding of difficulties, whether constitutional, developmental, or emotional, combined, say, with temporary ill-health, school absence or a change of class or school, certainly results in some boys attempting to hide their problems and to avoid reading. The longer this persists, and the more reading experience they miss, the more difficult it becomes for their parents and teachers to help them. Even finding suitable books on which to get them started is a problem, for they will often reject as "babyish" books appropriate to their reading ability. Having lost years of steady progress and of the experience of reading a wide variety of printed language, it is not surprising that their written language and their spelling will often lag even further behind.

One of the major challenges of remedial education is to provide these boys with accelerated programmes of reading experience which will enable them to develop their hard-won skill hand-in-hand with the mastery of efficient handwriting and the conventions of spelling. Too often these children are helped to learn to read and left to catch up on their own, very much as if, having learned the knack of swimming and demonstrated that they can perform a few strokes unsupported in the swimming pool, they can be safely dropped in the sea and will make it to the shore.

Are there signs by which we can identify dyslexic children?

The attempt to identify dyslexic children as a distinct group different from retarded or slow readers has led to two main lines of enquiry. The search for "hard" neurological evidence, such as the existence of lesions, tumours or incomplete cerebral development, has produced very few cases. Today we are unaware of any research which is concerned with identifying structural brain damage or malformation as a cause of dyslexia in children, apart from that concerned with acquired dyslexia or in association with other handicaps.

The other line of enquiry has been into the possibility that dyslexia may be associated with some form of "minimal brain damage" which may be identified by neurological "soft" signs such as clumsiness or jerky movements. Not only do the criteria by which these signs are assessed vary, but there is no agreement as to what signs or group of signs are significant. Children with a number of these "soft" signs usually have lower general levels of educational performance of which their reading difficulties are but one of the consequences.

There is evidence that perinatal complications such as prematurity or a "difficult" birth are associated with reading difficulties. In one study, 15% of children with two or more complications at birth were found to have reading difficulties. This, of course, fails to account for the percentage who had no reading difficulties and for those children who have reading difficulties but had no complications at birth. All one can say is that perinatal complications result in some children having reading difficulties.

Because no one "soft" neurological sign has been identified, research has attempted to identify groups of signs associated with dyslexia in children. Clusters of signs, syndromes, have been suggested, as have complex or variable syndromes. Complex or variable syndromes are groups of signs only some of which may be present in one child while another grouping of the signs may be present in another child.

One of the most frequent signs identified is that of difficulty in sequencing, whether it be remembering the days of the week after Wednesday, repeating a series of words or numbers (fox, bag, water, jam, path; 7,5,1,9,3) as given or in reverse order, or in reproducing in correct sequence a number of objects or shapes. Mirror writing and letter reversals, cross-laterality (being right-handed and left-eyed, for instance) and the inability to say which finger has been touched (finger agnosia) are among the many signs which have been associated with reading difficulties. Some of them warrant more detailed examination but it should be stated that not only is there no general agreement about their significance, it is also maintained that these syndromes can only be adequately diagnosed and assessed medically. Many of these signs are so common, however, that they have been recognized and assessed by remedial teachers and educational psychologists as possible factors in children's learning difficulties for many years. What is well established is that, without in any way denying that they may be significant factors in some children's difficulties, these signs are frequently present in substantial numbers of efficient readers. Certainly, what medical evidence there is has still to be established as being clinically predictive of reading difficulties.

The great value in having "soft" signs, could they be established, would be to enable whoever carried out pre-school examinations of children to identify those who would need special help in learning to read. It is in this sense that we say that, so far, none of the "signs" or complex, variable syndromes have clinically predictive value. Even when it can clearly be established that a child is lagging behind in speech development at age 4 years, has jerky movements, draws shapes back to front and is left-handed, right-eyed and right-footed, we doubt if anyone would be so foolhardy as to predict that she would be likely to have reading difficulties — without first of all finding out one simple basic fact: can she read already? In the present state of the art, it would be equally foolhardy to rely on these signs alone even were the child eight years of age.

What about laterality and cerebral dominance?

Laterality is our awareness of left and right and our preference for using one hand, eye, foot or ear rather than the other. Most people are right-handed, right-footed and use their right eyes and ears, should they be required to use only one, as, for instance, for looking through or listening at a keyhole. Estimates vary of the number of completely left-handed people from between 5 and 10% of the population. Some people, of course, are completely ambidextrous. Laterality develops during infancy and is, in part, associated with the fact that the left hemisphere of the brain usually assumes dominance for language and for skilled dexterity and movement.

But laterality is by no means a straightforward matter, nor is it fully understood! It does not follow that because right-handed people are usually left-hemisphere dominant, left-handed people are right-hemisphere dominant. In fact, two-thirds of left-handed people also have their language processing area in the left hemi-sphere. It is the anomalies of handedness which have long preoccupied those concerned with reading, writing and spelling difficulties. Children who are right-handed but left-eyed or left-footed, or vice versa, are said to be cross-lateral and there is evidence that cross-laterality may be associated with reading difficulties in some children. However, as many children who are cross-lateral are, in fact, efficient readers the concern about laterality has shifted to the investigation of cerebral dominance as a more significant and related factor.

Whereas laterality is concerned with our awareness of and preference for a particular hand, eye, ear or foot, cerebral dominance is used to describe the way in which one side of the brain assumes a specialized role for languge and higher cognitive processing. The two walnut-like halves of man's brain, as we have already remarked, are not equal in size. The left hemisphere is not only larger, but its surface, the cerebral cortex, is more deeply fissured and convoluted. All the evidence points to the fact that our brains may have the capacity to develop dominance in either hemisphere but that the left is better able to accommodate the specialized functions of language, finger dexterity and many higher cognitive functions including serial ordering. What does appear to cause difficulties, it is suggested, is unresolved dominance or an imbalance between the two hemispheres in language activities.

The right hemisphere's contribution to language is small but significant. But it is in its involvement in spatial orientation that it plays a major part in processing print. It is argued that when boys develop early spatial abilities, and when dominance has not been fully developed in the left hemisphere for language and for serial ordering essential for reading print, they are liable to have reading difficulties. They have been typified as having "two right hemispheres and no left". Girls develop language and, therefore, cerebral dominance, earlier than boys and, moreover, spatial orientation develops later than in boys. They are, developmentally, much less likely to have these reading difficulties, it is suggested.

Support for this theory is given by the fact that patients who have had the two hemispheres separated surgically have been shown to have difficulty in naming objects held in their left hands if they cannot see them. This demonstrates not only the role of the left hemisphere but also the importance of the connections between the hemispheres through the corpus callosum and the commissures, or bundles of nerve fibres. EEG studies, micro-electrodes and a number of modern techniques are being used to investigate both the functions of the right hemisphere, about which much less is known, and the interaction of the hemispheres.

Techniques have also been developed to study what happens when information is presented to the left and right eyes and ears separately. As part of the visual field of each eye is processed by the opposite hemisphere it is possible to compare differences in the responses of a subject to stimuli by each hemisphere independently. It is also possible to make comparisons between the responses of different subjects, such as those who are left handed and those who are right handed or between those who are efficient readers and those who are dyslexic. These "visual half-field" and "dichotic listening" tests, like other studies of laterality, however, have produced conflicting evidence. Some researchers have found differences between dyslexic children and able readers which, they argue, support the view that dominance has not been established in the dyslexic group. Other researchers have not found significant differences between the groups and point to the fact that many able readers exhibit the same characteristics on these tests as dyslexic children. It is difficult, therefore, to support the view that cerebral dominance and maturational lag in the case of boys are, in themselves, factors which account for these children's reading difficulties.

The evidence is similarly conflicting when research into the possibility that poor integration of what is seen with what is heard is a cause of reading difficulties. It has been argued that excessive neural activity in the right hemisphere, as evidenced by EEG studies, demonstrates that dyslexic boys are attending to the spatial aspects of print rather than to its serial ordering and to language. Other researchers have suggested that there is evidence that poor neural communication between the speech, visual and auditory centres of the brain is a cause of difficulties. Again, evidence is adduced to support the view that fatigue may set in on one channel of communication between the centres involved in reading. Clearly, it is essential in reading that information received by the eye is scanned efficiently, processed in the visual centre of the brain and communicated to the auditory and speech centres, so that what is read matches what has been heard which in turn will enable the reader to say the word. This cross-modal integration, as it is called, also involves memory of what has already been read and of language.

While the evidence remains inconclusive, and in some cases is dismissed completely, there is no doubt that inefficient processing of sight to sound to meaning, however or wherever it may arise, will make reading difficult. While inter-hemisphere transfer may or may not be a factor in dyslexic children's difficulties, inadequate attention to what is significant, and inadequate learning in any modality, whether in speech, visual or auditory perception, will cause difficulties. Perception, both visually and aurally, is a learned response to stimuli. We learn to judge distances and perspective, for example. Learning to read requires that we learn to attend to the significant cues of print.

One aspect of cerebral dominance is rarely mentioned, however.

There is research evidence to suggest that people who are right-hemisphere dominant have higher cognitive abilities than those who are left dominant. Such people are said to be better able to solve problems, think more divergently, integrate their thoughts with their emotions more successfully and meaningfully, and are generally more creative. Moreover, it is maintained, they are a misunderstood minority in a left-hemisphere dominant world. This is in complete contradistinction to those who would argue that dyslexic boys have "two right hermispheres and none left".

The problem of laterality and of cerebral dominance has to be seen against the background of human diversity and in the context of a brain which is not only involved in processing but in our levels of arousal and awareness, and in our planning and monitoring of our mental activities. We need both hemispheres, of that we can be sure. We need diversity and individual differences. Genetic inheritance is coded to ensure uniqueness. And we need more than one eye, one ear, one hand and one foot. While we are quite sure of the value and of the significance of the differences identified as being associated with some children's reading problems, we are also sure that in the majority of cases these difficulties, if they are developmental, will not persist, and if they are permanent, as in the case of cross-laterality or "crossed-hemisphere dominance", can be overcome by efficient learning. We recall visiting a school and discussing the laterality problems of a group of retarded readers with their teacher. Then we saw their fingers, in the next lesson. They were playing their recorders dextrously, ambidextrously and sweetly. "Had we been right?" we wondered. We still only have a tiny keyhole into the complexities of the brain.

Are reading difficulties associated with speech problems and with delayed speech development?

There is a substantial amount of evidence which confirms that some children with speech defects have developmental dyslexia or retardation in reading. Their speech problems are most commonly with the motor and physical processes of speech involved in articulation, but a wide range of speech problems, including substitutions of one sound for another, stumbling over words, and stuttering have been found to be associated with reading problems in some children. Children with marked speech defects at age seven years were found to be backward in reading at sixteen years. Many studies, including large-scale ones, confirm that children who are significantly late in acquiring speech are often poor readers and have difficulties with spelling. Speech problems and delayed development of speech are so commonly associated with reading difficulties that many researchers into dyslexia exclude this group of children from their samples. Many speech therapists, however, rightly consider that this group of "at risk" children need early identification and help if both their speech and reading difficulties are to be resolved. As speech therapy is concerned with the defects in the context of the children's language development the professional involvement of speech therapists in the area of reading difficulties is to be welcomed. Unfortunately, many children with speech defects and language difficulties are neither identified nor treated because of the shortage of speech therapists. There is substantial evidence that where children receive early therapy and where speech therapists involve parents and teachers in helping their children, considerable improvements can be made in reading.

Do hearing problems cause reading difficulties?

Deaf children have difficulties in the acquisition of all language skills, although a great deal naturally depends on whether or not they were born deaf and upon the age at which they became deaf. Reading may also be retarded by partial hearing-loss. High-frequency loss may prevent children from hearing or from distinguishing between many consonants; whereas low-frequency loss will impair their ability to distinguish vowel sounds. However, these more obvious difficulties are well understood and need not concern us here. They serve to highlight, however, the processing problems some children have with aural information.

Some children's reading difficulties have been associated with poor auditory discrimination, poor memory for what is heard, poor association of what is heard with what is printed, or poor cross-modal integration between what is heard and what is experienced through the other senses. Quite apart from those aspects of this problem which we discussed earlier, it has been suggested that, as with visual perceptual problems, some of these difficulties arise from a failure to develop selective attention to what is heard. Whether or not this is constitutionally determined or is the result of developmental lag or environmental factors, such as a noisy urban environment or a noisy and undemanding home, is open to question. "Central deafness" which is difficult to detect as it is a neural processing and not a physiological malfunction of the ear, is also thought to cause reading difficulties. A simple method of identifying central deafness has been developed in Canada and is now being used in England and Wales. One environmental aspect of hearing difficulties in young children is that of intermittent deafness caused by "glue-ear" and hearing loss caused by colds and other infections. Neither the children nor their parents and teachers may be aware of what is wrong unless or until something alerts them to it. These periods of temporary hearing loss, should they occur when children are acquiring language or learning to read, may well cause confusion, difficulty in distinguishing between words, in associating what they mis-hear with what they see, and an inability to discriminate voices from background noise. When hearing returns to normal the children may have a further period of confusion which again interferes with learning. They are in a similar situation to the experimenters who, having removed the lenses which turned the world upside down, must wait for the brain to reprocess visual information the right way up. If, when these children have resolved their difficulties, they experience another episode of impaired hearing, confusion may well be compounded. Their uncertainty further exacerbates their learning difficulties. We mention this problem because it is one which is frequently met in schools and because it demonstrates the importance of looking for feasible, simple explanations rather than remote ones to account for difficulties.

Are dyslexic children likely to have behaviour problems?

Definitions of dyslexia usually exclude emotional and behavioural problems as a cause of the reading difficulties and many researchers exclude from their samples children with these problems. However, not only is there substantial evidence which links emotional and behavioural problems with backwardness in school work and in reading, there is also considerable evidence which shows a higher incidence of these problems in poor readers than in good readers. In other words, difficulties in reading may be the cause of emotional and behaviour problems in some children, while these problems may cause other children to be retarded in reading. Our concern here is with those children who are failing in reading and who have no previous history of behavioural or emotional problems. The evidence suggests that some of these children may well develop emotional and behaviour problems.

The ability to read in young children is a socially desirable skill. It is an accomplishment expected of children by their parents, teachers and their peers, a milestone in development and thus a status symbol. Some children who fail to learn to read will accept the fact, possibly think it does not matter very much, and be sufficiently robust to brush aside the concern of parents and teachers or the scorn of their peers. Others will over-react: they will cope with their failure with bravado, seek attention and popularity in clowning or bullying, try to bluff their way through school and reject their parents' admonishments with defiance and displays of self-assertion. They are the easiest to identify with their attention-seeking behaviours, and the easiest to understand and to help.

Some children, however, try to hide. They make themselves as inconspicuous as possible, avoid situations in which their failure will be exposed, feel guilty and inadequate and turn in upon themselves. One study found that 10% of retarded readers were below average in aggression and showed excessive acceptance of self-blame. This compares with 4% who showed marked anti-social behaviours and hostility towards both adults and other children. Boys who are retarded in reading are more than twice as likely to show anxiety and lack of concentration, and three times as likely to experience irrational fears when compared with other children.

These behavioural and emotional problems of children with reading difficulties become particularly prevalent around the age of nine and are, need we say it, more common in boys than in girls. This suggests that neither the behaviours nor the reading difficulties have been recognized or dealt with early enough. The comforting assumption that both behaviour and reading difficulties are the result of a developmental lag should not absolve us of the responsibility of intervening to help these children. There is a body of evidence which shows that helping children with their behavioural problems often leads to an improvement in their reading, and that helping children with their reading problems often results in an improvement in their behaviours. The corollary is that the wise parent or teacher will do both. This requires sensitivity and skill. Above all it demands a respect for the children's integrity and a concern to enhance their self-image. Too often remedial reading may mean little more than finding out what the children can't do — and giving them a hell of a lot of it. This kind of remedial "help" has been likened to throwing a drowning man both ends of the rope!

If parents, as we have suggested earlier, by their interest and encouragement, play such a vital role in their children's progress in reading, it follows that some parents may have the opposite effect. Many researchers have indicated that reading difficulties are associated with primary emotional and behavioural disorders which are caused by poor parent–child relationships. Almost every type of inadequate parental behaviour has been nominated as a major contributor to these difficulties. Dominating, demanding, over-protective, rejecting, lacking in affection and passive parents have all been said to create behaviour problems in their children which lead to reading problems. Parents may not be able to change their personalities but most, once aware of distress in their children, can change their behaviour towards them. Others need early help and support. While we recognize the complexities of these parental and familial situations it is also important to recognize that they underline the importance of the contribution teachers can make by their influence, encouragement, support, counselling and, perhaps above all, their professional skills in helping children to enjoy security and success in learning to read, write and spell.

The child who has deep-seated and intractable reading difficulties, whether or not he is labelled dyslexic, is certainly vulnerable and may well have some permutation of the emotional and behavioural characteristics we have described. He will feel he is a failure, will usually be frustrated and perplexed by his difficulties, and feel either different from his peers or alienated from them. Many dyslexic and reading retarded children have commented upon the effect this has upon their ability to make and keep friends, an important component of growing up. Frequently, although it may be well disguised, they have a poor self-image. They know that basically they are as good and as worthy as anyone else but they none the less have low self-esteem: other kids can read but they can't. Without early help, if their reading and emotional and behavioural difficulties are allowed to persist, there is a high risk that between the ages of eight and eleven there will be a progressive deterioration in their behaviour. Fortunately, some children are remarkably resilient, but for all of them reading difficulties are like deafness in that there is no external sign that anything is wrong: the children carry the problem inside them all the time.

Do dyslexic children have handwriting problems or do mirror writing?

That some children have writing problems and write letters and words the wrong way round in addition to their reading difficulties is not in doubt. Some dyslexic children show a preference for reading print when it is upside-down. A variety of explanations have been put forward for mirror writing and it was extensively investigated by Dr Samuel Orton in America from the mid-1920s. He conceptualized word-blindness as strephosymbolia, or twisted symbols, caused not by a neurological defect but by a peculiarity of brain organization. This he believed to be the result of faulty communication of the visual "image" from the right to the left hemisphere. He advocated that children should be helped by using the sense of touch to establish the correct orientation of letters and words.

Another explanation is that there is a "writing centre" in the dominant hemisphere but a memory for writing movements in both hemispheres. It is suggested that, in cases of unresolved dominance, the child copies the reversed "image" from the hemisphere not involved in the act of writing. Cerebral dominance and laterality is used to support a third explanation which argues that our most natural movements are from the centre-line of the body outwards. Thus the right-handed write from left to right. The left-handed would find it more natural to write from right to left. In two-handed operations we find it easier when one hand mirrors the activity of the other, it is suggested. Thus, a right-handed person, required to write with both hands simultaneously, would write a mirror image with the left hand of whatever was being written by the right. From this, it is deduced that mirror writers are really people who would have found it easier had they adopted the left hand as the preferred hand.

As mirror writing is common in beginning writers, the persistence of mirror writing is also attributed to maturational lag: the children are slow to develop the neural processes appropriate to representing what they see with what they write. A more convincing and simpler explanation is that mirror writing is a 'generalized' response in beginning writers: they copy the shape correctly but ignore its orientation. With some letters such as A, H, I, M, O, T or o, m, w, x, they will be right in any case, but with others, such as a, h, t or E, R, P they would be wrong. The chances are, however, that unless they are detected and corrected, many of them will also be forming all their letters from right to left, in other words backwards. Failure to detect that children are not only reversing some letters but forming others with the wrong directional sequence of strokes, results in them reinforcing and learning an inappropriate strategy. In other words, they are efficiently learning a bad habit. As bad habits can take as long to unlearn as it takes to learn good habits these children are doubly disadvantaged. Fortunately, techniques such as those developed by Grace Fernald, which we will discuss later, are usually successful in correcting mirror writing and letter reversals.

Although poor handwriting is often associated with dyslexia as one of its characteristics the problem is most readily accounted for by the fact that the children are uncertain and confused about how to encode language in writing. If they can't read it, they can't write it. They are not helped by the fact that the written letters are variants of their printed forms e.g. A, a, *a, A, a*. Nor are they helped by sitting a long way from a blackboard copying white letters on to white paper with black pencils. Perhaps many children are most ill-served by being required to read what someone else has written down out of his head before they have learned how to write down what was in their own heads. Whether or not parents and teachers subscribe to a language-experience approach to reading they will help these children most if they teach the skills of reading, writing and spelling "hand-in-hand".

Do dyslexic children have poor memories?

"Glynn's got a marvellous memory — except for reading," explained his mother., "He seems to forget whatever he's learned quicker than it took him to learn it!" Glynn's mother identified a characteristic both of many children with reading difficulties and of memory itself. Although memory is a general characteristic of mental activity it is specific to particular processes. We may have a good memory for faces but a bad one for names, a good memory for places but a bad one for telephone numbers. In the classroom we recognize the difference between children who have good visual memories and those who have good auditory ones. In the laboratory we may distinguish, too, between differences in the reception, retention, recognition and recall of what is being learned. Thus, Glynn may have retained a memory of what he had learned but have been unable to recall it. The many attributes of memory have been studied since the beginnings of psychology but how memories are laid down, stored and retrieved in the brain is still not fully understood. It is now thought that memory traces are changes in RNA levels in nerve cells and their surrounding glia but we are a long way from understanding the biochemistry of memory's complex processes or all its tricks.

Although it is known that some lesions to the brain can cause severe disturbances of memory, there is no neurological explanation which satisfactorily accounts for children's memory difficulties in learning to read. Most of the research has concentrated upon those aspects of the reading process which involve specific types of memory such as short-term memory, visual memory, verbal memory, auditory memory and sequential memory. In all of these areas there is research which suggests that dyslexic children are defective in one or more of them.

This has led other researchers to suggest that dyslexic children's difficulties are not accounted for by memory deficits but from an inability to attend to the significant characteristics of words, letters, sounds, sequences or meaning. We suspect that they are both right and that what they are describing are learning difficulties. All perception is a matter of learning to make the right guesses about the significance, relevance or meaning of the information we receive through our senses.

In the box below are four similar signs.

1	2	3	4

Asked to identify the "odd one out" the reader's likely reaction would be to say that they are all the same.

Pressed further, one might well refer to the gap in the corner of Sign 1 or to the fact that the second stroke in Sign 4 is not in the middle. A Russian reader would immediately recognize Sign 2 as the "odd man out", as the letter for the sound "shch" in a row of letters for the sound "sh". For the Russian, the tiny tail extending from the final stroke is as significant as the difference between "c" and "e". But even when we know what to attend to, everything depends on the circumstances under which we wish to recall information. We all know the days of the week but, it has been said, trying to repeat them from memory in alphabetical order is likely to induce confusional amnesia!

Given the need, we can respond to stimuli almost immediately. This suggests that there is some sensory memory involved into which information is coded and retained long enough for it to be dealt with or dismissed. If necessary this sensory memory can retain information for up to about 2,000 milliseconds while its features are examined. However, when we run our eyes down the names in a telephone directory, for instance, we can hold information for up to about 30 seconds while we examine it. This memory is commonly called Short Term Memory. It lasts long enough to read a telephone number and dial it, say, but if we need to retain the number it must be coded into Long Term Memory where it may remain and be recalled minutes or even years later. Recent research retains these distinctions, for they describe how we think our memory behaves, but suggests that instead of Sensory or Immediate, Short Term and Long Term Memory, each with different Stores, there is a Primary Memory and a long term memory designated Secondary Memory. Certainly the relationships between visual, auditory and other sensory or Primary Memories, on the one hand, and between them and Secondary or Long Term Memory, must be very flexible. When we read, as we have seen in Chapter 3, we are able, apparently simultaneously, to recognize the print, process it visually, code it into the auditory and semantic memory, transfer the code to the speech area and articulate what we have read. We retain the meaning of what we have read, possibly its position on a page, but we rarely retain in memory an image of print on the page or of the sound of our voice. In proficient reading, then, efficient recognition and coding of print, together with efficient transfer of the coded information from one sensory processing area to another, each apparently with a memory which recognizes and sifts what is important, are all involved. But at any stage Long Term or Secondary Memory may be brought in if we need it, as for example, if we do not immediately *recognize* the name of a character introduced earlier in a book we are reading.

Some evidence supports the view that dyslexic children and poor readers need a longer time to process visual information than do efficient readers. Other research has not found this difference. Attentional levels have also been found to be a factor and it is possible that poor visual recognition of letters, phonemes or words, combined with uncertainty about their sounds or meanings, militate against some children learning to read. Similarly, as Primary or Short Term Memory has a limited storage capacity of about seven bits of information, it is argued that dyslexic children are defective in recognizing economic ways of coding print. For example, given three nonsense words, FUV, PUM, KUX, they will attempt to remember them as nine letters, whereas the efficient reader only has to remember three 'words', *fuv, pum, kux*. Certainly, the more strategies we have for coding information when we see it, attend to it and transfer it, the more efficiently we process it. Dyslexics have been found to be as good as able readers at remembering simple shapes and even Hebrew letters and words with which they were not previously familiar. But they were not as good at remembering nonsense words. This in turn suggests that they have not poor memories but are defective in verbal coding and verbal memory.

In this connection it is interesting to note that in Czechoslovakia, which has a phonetically consistent alphabet with each letter always having the same sound, dyslexic children's difficulties are not so much with this verbal coding into sound units. There the children have difficulty in breaking words up into syllables. Thus LISTOPAD (November) is LIST/O-PAD and not LI/STOP/AD or LIS/TOP/AD. Remediation concentrates not merely upon focusing attention upon the syllables but in helping children to understand that the syllables often have a meaning. LIST(leaf) + OPAD(fall) = the month when leaves fall. In English-speaking countries teachers are increasingly giving attention to the meaningful elements, the morphemes, in remedial programmes. Unfortunately, not having a phonetically consistent alphabet ("ieu" = "ef" or "oo" as in "lieutenant"), our children cannot escape some mastery of the main phonemes too. But they need to know only the main characteristics, not all the irregularities and exceptions. Context and meaning tell us more than the letter shapes or clusters.

Some dyslexic children have been found to have no problems with the recall of visual information but to have difficulties in recalling auditory information, such as a sequence of taps with a pencil on a table (.. ... .). This ability is involved in syllabification, in the recognition of the rhythmic pattern of words and language. Combined with poor ability to "chunk" visual information it is understandable that there might be a deficiency in remembering the sound of the word and its printed form. Thus, inadequate coding in auditory memory, together with poor coding of print into visual memory, prevent it from being coded into semantic (meaning of words) memory. This may well be a component in the failure of "cross-modal integration" previously discussed. In reading, the more strategies we have for sorting and sifting language the fewer the demands made upon memory and the more efficiently we will "guess" the meaning. Only when the efficient reader meets an unfamiliar word or phrase is it necessary to pause and refer to Secondary or Long Term Memory.

Secondary or Long Term Memory contains all that we know and think we have forgotten until we find we can recall it! In it is the deep structure of language. The strategies available to us for accessing all that is in its store are infinitely more subtle and complex than those of Primary or Short Term Memory. For the richness of its store, and our ability to find what we want in it, derives largely from our facility with language, whether that language be that of our mother and other tongues, the language of mathematics, sciences, symbols or music. Our facility in language is the result of efficient coding, classifying, naming and interrelating both during and after encoding in Primary or Short Term Memory. This is evidenced when we read a paragraph in a newspaper and subsequently tell someone about what we read.

Efficient naming and labelling facilitates both storage and retrieval from memory. It is in naming and labelling that some dyslexic children have been found to be deficient. They have been found by some researchers to be slow at naming letters, objects, colours and pictures. This, in turn, makes for difficulties in retrieval, very much as if a piece of correspondence were filed but, instead of being coded alphabetically according to the correspondent's name or classified according to its subject matter, it had been put in the filing cabinet at random. Now poorly coded visual information, poorly "chunked" auditory information, to which it has been poorly coded, has been poorly labelled and classified in Secondary or Long Term Memory. Not surprisingly, when Glynn sees the book next day, all he remembers is the colour of its cover.

Further research has shown that some dyslexic children are poor at retaining complex information over a period of time and, if the material was printed in the first case, this is not surprising. Few of the children most researchers have encountered exhibit an overall deficiency in memory. But there is considerable agreement that many dyslexic children have difficulty in remembering sequential series such as their tables or months of the year. They have been found to be particularly defective in remembering sequences of letters and words and tasks which involve verbal information. This includes tasks in which, as we have seen, memorization may be helped by saying the names of objects or numbers, by encoding them verbally. There is supportive evidence for this in the performance of some of these children in sub-tests and items in "intelligence" tests. Thus a child who fails to encode a series of numbers verbally (7 9 3 0 4 5 1 as 'seven, nine, three, zero, four, five, one') may have greater difficulty in repeating them in reverse order than one who does. This evidence suggests a deficit or developmental lag in auditory memory.

The research into memory deficits of dyslexic children is significant in that it not only supports Glynn's mother's observation but also alerts us to the complexity of memory coding and processing. It is by no means conclusive and is limited by our lack of understanding of memory save at a schematic psychological level. Take away the concepts of Immediate, Short and Long Term Memory and their 'stores', and replace them with biochemical changes in the neurons which are changed according to the intensity or frequency of their stimuli and we might reasonably conceptualize the process as *learning*. Certainly, the difficulty in constructing tests of memory is that we can rarely be sure whether we are testing memory or testing what the person knows already; and we can never do this satisfactorily because how we perceive is how we have learned to perceive. This is consonant with modern theories of memory which distinguish only between Primary Memory and Secondary Memory. Perhaps the biggest function of Primary Memory is forgetting, the extinction of all the transient and irrelevant stimuli our senses receive, so that our brains retain the capacity to process those which have the highest significance or survival value. Its second most valuable attribute is that of recognition, its ability to be sensitive to the essential, minimal characteristics or stimuli, whether verbal, visual, auditory, spatial, semantic or tactile, which it has learned from experience are significant. Children with reading difficulties, as we have seen, have not adequately learned these discriminatory strategies. In some children it may well be that visual memory of letters and words is defective, in others it may well be that auditory memory is poor.

Those children who cannot recall reversed sequences of numbers or signs, or who cannot adequately relate what they have seen with what they have heard, may be deficient in the coding and review strategies of Primary Memory. It is doubtful, however, if these children have a deficiency in memory as such, as in every other respect they demonstrably perform normally. Many of them are highly verbal and it is their general ability which highlights their reading and spelling problems. It is only in the encoding and decoding of language into and from print that they have difficulty in remembering. This suggests that their problems are learning difficulties, particularly in the perceptual processes of Primary Memory. They have not learned to perceive the right things. This view is supported by the fact that, as we shall see later when we discuss remedial methods, given the right help to increase their repertoire of coding skills and to recognize what is significant in the surface structure of language, they can learn to read. However, these strategies must be integrated with all the array of the strategies of Secondary Memory, that is, integrated with the meaning of language in which the majority are by no means deficient. They must learn to look for meaning.

Do dyslexic children have erratic eye movements?

Until recently all the research has concentrated upon what goes on "behind the eyes" of dyslexic children. An entirely different approach has investigated what goes on *in* the eyes of children with reading difficulties.

When we read, our eyes do not scan the lines of print in smooth sweeps. Rather, our eyes move in short, grasshopper jerks or jumps. These are called saccadic eye movements. It has been shown that dyslexic children, when given carefully designed clinical tests, have abnormal saccadic eye movements. Unlike proficient readers, their saccadic movements are short and erratic. What is considered to be particularly significant is that the backward jumps, which are normally short, are much longer in dyslexic children. Whether or not these erratic eye-movements are constitutional or developmental remains to be determined. Again, it is still not clear whether or not they are the result, rather than the cause, of the reading difficulties. This research is important because it, too, like the research into their memorizing difficulties, underlines the importance of developing economic and efficient scanning of visual information. If erratic saccadic eye-movements are the cause of dyslexia in some children then, for the first time, it may be possible to identify and correct them before children start learning to read.

Is dyslexia the result of a language deficiency?

Whatever research one examines in connection with reading difficulties the question must always be asked, "What or how does it relate to language?" Dyslexic children may have crossed-laterality, poor cerebral dominance or get easily fatigued, but so do many efficient readers. As we have seen, many researchers have countered the claims of other researchers by demonstrating that, in their samples of children, this has been the case. Again, if the children have been selected by carefully excluding pupils with other defects or disabilities, so that researchers are left with children whose abilities are "normal" in every respect save in their reading difficulties, would it not be prudent to look carefully at their language abilities?

Researchers have, therefore, investigated selected samples of dyslexic children to determine whether or not they have a language deficit or exhibit deficiencies in language abilities which might account for their reading problems. Some researchers have found that the children they have studied have attentional defects, in that they fail to give selective attention to the various cues which help them gain meaning from print. In addition, however, they found that the children had limited vocabularies, had poor ability to infer the meanings of words from their contexts, lacked understanding of the relationship between spoken and written words and language, and had an inadequate knowledge of syntax — the way words go together in sentences. They suggest that it is these inherent deficits in language which are at the root of the children's reading problems.

This research is supported by the evidence of other researchers concerned with the difficulties of children whose cultural and language disadvantages are a factor in learning to read. But the link has to be regarded as a tenuous one. Linguistically deprived children and children for whom English is a second language, given appropriate education which compensates them for their linguistic deficiencies in oral English and given instruction in reading, not only learn to read: reading plays a major part in developing their knowledge and understanding of the structure and nuances of language. The history of education demonstrates how rapidly illiteracy and semi-literacy can be reduced in populations, given the right incentives and appropriate opportunities. The large numbers of pupils in our schools and of students in our universities who have had to learn English and to read and write, often with the minimum of help, during the early years of schooling, are evidence that language deficiencies are not an insuperable barrier to learning to read. That these deficiencies create difficulties is not in doubt. That they are at the root of otherwise able and competent children's difficulties is extremely implausible. If they are a factor in combination with other difficulties, it can only be assumed that they are secondary.

A more reasonable explanation of these children's deficiencies is that they are the result of their lack of reading experience. Learning to read makes us aware of language. As we discussed earlier, reading develops consciousness of words in a linear order in contradistinction to the temporal order of speech. Because, in written language, we have no situational, environmental cues to meaning, the language of print must provide its own context. Syntax must be more precise and particular. Reading both requires and develops consciousness of the richness and subtlety of vocabulary, of the variety of functions of words, and of the complexities of the structure of language. Children who cannot read and who have not read widely have been denied this experience. Their sense of failure and inadequacy will, in turn, add to their uncertainties about the nature of language and its use. But the fact that some children have these difficulties, which is not denied, and also have difficulties in learning to read, fails to explain why many children who have no language deficits find reading difficult.

Do dyslexic children have persistent spelling difficulties?

We have already referred to research associated with the problems some children have with spelling but this question frequently arises because many definitions of dyslexia include reference to both erratic spelling and to persistent spelling difficulties after the children have learned to read.

Researchers have identified a variety of common types of error made by dyslexic children. Bizarre spelling which shows no relation to the sound or shape of words is rare and the majority of errors are reversals of letter sequences, substitutions of letter clusters by inappropriate ones, and phonetic errors. The most perplexing errors are, of course, the bizarre ones and these may well occur even when the child is merely copying. Many children who make this kind of error also have extremely poor handwriting so that it is almost impossible to decipher what they have written. However, bizarre spelling sometimes occurs in association with perfectly executed handwriting. Bizarre spelling has been accounted for by a deficiency in the lexical encoding ability of dyslexic children: they are slow to distinguish between the different sounds of words; slow to distinguish written letters, letter groups and words; slow to relate sounds of letters and words to their printed forms; they take a long time to learn visually or auditorily presented information; they have poor memories for what they have learned whether visually, auditorily or both. All of these difficulties indicate that the children have problems in the recognition and the processing of langauge in its symbolic form and this is borne out by the fact that, certainly in so far as reading, writing and spelling are concerned, they are best helped by concrete cues and by a multisensory approach which employs the sense of touch together with strong and clear visual and auditory impressions. As we have already indicated, poor intersensory processing of language in its spoken and printed forms, whether the result of maturational lag, unresolved cerebral dominance, lack of language consciousness or of memory deficits, is somewhere at the heart of these children's difficulties.

The more common errors many children make in spelling, such as reversals of letters and clusters, and substitutions of inappropriate phonic constructions (*ruf* for *rough*), are more readily accounted for. In part they are problems of attention to serial ordering and to sight–sound–sense correspondence, in part the result of the children's limited experience of the printed and written forms of language, and in part the result of the apparent inconsistencies of English spelling. Far too much is made of the latter. While there is no denying that our orthography is at times confusing, it also contains a core of considerable consistency. Moreover, many of the apparent inconsistencies are the result of the incorporation in our language of words from Greek, Latin and other languages, to which we have already referred, and the preservation of some of the conventions of those languages' orthography, or of approximations to them, which reflect their origins and provide cues to meaning and appropriateness. Some people are fortunate to assimilate spelling with little conscious effort but most of us either need to be taught it or to make an effort to learn it. Too much is also made of the persistent spelling difficulties some children have when they have at last learned to read. We have seen some doctoral theses on the subject with such complexes of complex spelling rules that we could only assume the dyslexic pupils, for whom they were designed, would have to take higher degrees themselves before they understood them. Finally, too much is made of spelling mistakes by both parents and teachers simply because they are the easiest to notice and to mark with a single stroke. This tendency persists in much of the literature concerned with dyslexia and suggests that there is an assumption that everyone spells correctly all of the time and that spelling errors betoken some regrettable fall from grace. The letters which newspaper offices, headteachers and education offices receive daily, from all strata of society, indicate that for many people spelling has been neither caught nor taught. But that some people find spelling a persistent problem cannot be denied.

Conclusions

The research literature suggests that there is no single characteristic of dyslexia other than a difficulty with reading. The difficulty with reading may have a variety of causes and a variety of manifest-ations. Attempts to explain these difficulties are limited by our limited knowledge of cerebral processes and are frequently specu-lative. That the difficulties exist, however, is not in doubt.

What does emerge from the literature is that different children have different difficulties and that little purpose is served by labelling them as a discrete category. It is also clear that reading is a complex cognitive ability and that any analysis of children's diffi-culties in acquiring it must be concerned to identify in which specific process or processes of the complex of processes their difficulties may lie. If their difficulties are with sequential ordering, cross-modal integration, with visual or auditory or semantic memory, with spelling or with writing, then far better that they should be so described. Lumping them together as reading diffi-culties is equally vague and misleading. It is even more vague and misleading to describe the difficulties as specific learning difficulties. This begs even more questions and may deflect us from discerning the true nature of these children's needs in specific aspects of the process of reading.

The research so far has alerted us to the existence of the problems in all their diversity. The way forward for research must be towards greater specificity, more rigorous research design and research in much greater depth. Above all, in place of speculation and global conclusions from a modicum of evidence, there is a great need for wielding Occam's Razor, the principle that entities should not be multiplied beyond necessity, and for parismony and economy in the design and interpretation of research evidence. Instead of seeking explanations in their neuro-biology we should first seek explanations in the children's on-task performance in reading.

Parents and teachers are usually not directly involved with these concerns. But they, too, in the light of the research evidence we have briefly examined, may well wonder what its implications are for them. We suggest that, in the absence of any agreed research evidence as to the cause and nature of the children's difficulties, they would be far better advised to forego the use of terms such as dyslexia — and to tell it as it is. Instead of begging questions, to which no one has an adequate answer and which may involve them in fruitless discussion, all they need say is what they know. "Pat's having difficulty with reading — she can't even read her little brother's books, and she's nearly twelve." "William is illiterate. He's nine and still doesn't know his letters. Unless I tell him, he holds his book the wrong way up." "Margaret is eight and she's still struggling to read the books she had when she started school. Her spelling and writing are atrocious, too." Comments such as these, which are factual and immediately comprehensible, say far more than trading labels such as dyslexia, dysgraphia or poorly established cerebral dominance. And they are far more likely to get action, too. Teachers may prefer to call their descriptions "criterion references" and give more detailed descriptions of their children's reading and other abilities. It is, we suggest, far better to let the experts choose their own labels if they still persist in using them. Some may even mutter things like Gerstmann Syndrome or narremic substitutions. The shibboleths they use will undoubtedly be the keys to their own particular box of assessment and diagnostic tests they use to examine the nature of the children's reading difficulties. In the last analysis what matters is how accurately they can assess the children's special educational needs and how effectively they can meet them. Like the millions of illiterate and semiliterate children in the world, these children have not had adequate and appropriate incentives and opportunities to learn to read which were sufficiently in harmony with their developing powers. How their needs are assessed, and how they are met, we will examine in the following chapters.

CHAPTER 6

Reasons and Remedies — Assessment, Diagnosis and Remediation

"One finger in the throat and one in the rectum make a good diagnostician." Sir William Osler

Identifying children with reading difficulties presents few problems. Whether in the family or the classroom, their failure when others are succeeding proclaims them. What is problematic is to identify them early enough and to determine why they are failing and how to help them to succeed.

In the vast majority of cases of reading difficulty the reasons are not hard to find. Environmental factors such as poor housing, inadequate diet, lack of sleep, general neglect and cultural deprivation account for many children's reading difficulties. Constitutional factors such as low general ability, sensory defects of sight and hearing, respiratory and speech disorders may frequently give rise to problems in learning to read. Emotional and behavioural difficulties, poor social adjustment and the effects of family turbulence, whether caused by frequent changes of home in service families, matrimonial stress or familial bereavements and illness, are also common factors.

Often, however, despite the vigilance of parents, medical, social and education services, it is only when children start to learn to read that some problems come to the surface. Intermittent deafness resulting from colds is frequently first noticed in the classroom. Visual defects, too, may be first observed when children peer at their books or come to the front of the class to read the board. In one

114

research project in which we were involved, out of 350 seven-year-olds, all of whom had previously been medically examined, 10% were found to have defects of sight or hearing. Children and their needs are changing all the time. Experienced teachers can usually list hundreds of obvious and bizarre reasons for children's reading difficulties which they have encountered with beginning readers. Cases like Tristram, a healthy ball of fire at home, who in the classroom couldn't sit still and was more like a ball *on* fire; Pat, sweet, compliant, shy and a dreamer to her parents, seemed to her teacher to have times when she was "absent", fugues which made the doctor suspect *petit mal* but which he found to be caused by a quirk of Pat's blood-sugar metabolism; or Mark who burst into tears when asked to read and whose mother said he was just like her, "a bag of nerves", but was later found to be badly bruised on his arms and back where father had been beating reading into him. Many teachers could fill a case-book of such reasons for reading and other difficulties. And many can justifiably claim they have never met a problem they couldn't lick from their own resources or with the help of doctors, psychologists or therapists.

It is only when we have eliminated all possible reasons that we occasionally find children with difficulties which we still cannot account for. They are extremely rare and often parents and teachers persist in searching for reasons and trying to overcome the difficulties. If they have the time and a repertoire of skills they may well succeed. If they haven't, they may well consider the children should be assessed and the reasons for the difficulties diagnosed.

Multidisciplinary assessment

In both North America and the UK, educational legislation recognizes that children with disabilities or learning difficulties have special educational needs for which special educational provision should be made. In some form or another, most states in the USA, the provinces of Canada, Scotland, England and Wales require that, in order that the education provided should match the needs of the children, an assessment should be made of their needs by doctors, psychologists and their schools. This multidisciplinary assessment, for instance, is a requirement of the 1981 Education Act in England and Wales. Under the Act, local education authorities must notify the parents, the social services and district health authorities, and seek advice concerning the educational, medical and psychological or other features of the cases which they consider relevant to the children's present and future educational needs. The professionals consulted may consult such others they consider it expedient or advisable to consult and the education authority must take into consideration any representations made by the parents. This comprehensive assessment enables the education authority to specify the children's special educational needs and to make a statement setting out the provisions it considers appropriate to meet them. The special educational provisions include: the type of school or particular school considered appropriate; any additional provision such as, say, speech therapy, or support by the social services; and other provisions considered desirable for the children to benefit from the special educational provisions.

Whether described as dyslexic, severely reading retarded or having a specific learning difficulty in reading by parents, teachers or specialists is irrelevant at the stage at which a child is considered for assessment, so far as this Act is concerned. What is relevant is that the child "has a significantly greater difficulty in learning than the majority of children of his age" or "has a disability which either prevents or hinders him from making use of educational facilities of a kind generally provided in schools". A child who is failing at reading and has not responded to such remedial teaching as is generally provided may properly be considered as included in the provisions of the Act.

The doctor's role

Although the British Medical Association has advised doctors that, because specific developmental dyslexia is not susceptible to medical diagnosis, it should be assessed by educational psychologists, it does not follow that doctors will not examine cases of dyslexia or severe reading difficulties in children. Medical advice will still be sought to determine whether there are sensory, physical, neurological or other defects, disabilities or handicaps which affect the children's ability to learn and benefit from education. Under the Act, moreover, doctors can request such specialist advice as they consider advisable so that they may, if they wish, request, say, a neurological or ophthalmological investigation.

The psychologist's role

The Educational Psychologists' role is central to the assessment of reading difficulties. Assessment is regarded by them as the systematic collection of all the relevant data about a child, organizing that data, analysing it, and then making the best possible prediction of what will best bring about the desired changes in the child. In looking at children, they will not only try to get as clear a picture as possible of the children themselves but also of their situation in the family, in their relations with others and in the school.

Tests of ability

Educational psychologists commonly include in their assessments tests of ability and performance and, although they are often accused of testing intelligence, most would deny this! The tests they use are batteries of sub-tests of a wide range of abilities such as the WISC (Wechsler Intelligence Scale for Children), the Terman-Merrill revision of the Stanford Binet test, and the BAS (British Ability Scales). These are individually administered tests, as opposed to the group tests of verbal or non-verbal abilities which are used in schools for coarse-screening large numbers of pupils. These tests, with the exception of the BAS, were originally designed as intelligence tests. Because they have all been standardized on large numbers of children and cover a wide spectrum of abilities, they enable psychologists both to compare a child's abilities with the norms for his or her age and to compare how a child is functioning is, say, comprehension and general knowledge or vocabulary and coding. In fact most psychologists regard the tests as structured interviews which provide reliable data to be analysed in the context of all the other data, rather than just a means of arriving at a score of ability, performance or intelligence.

But whatever reservations individual psychologists may have about these tests in their general application, all of them have difficulty when it comes to interpreting the results when investigating reading problems. This is because it is impossible to determine the extent to which the results reflect not so much the children's abilities as their reading difficulties which have deprived them of language and educational experience. All these tests reflect, in part, the children's experience and these children have been missing a vital part of it. Again, as some of the sub-tests may be testing skills and subskills involved in reading, the children's scores may be further depressed. Coding, which is a sub-test of the WISC, for instance, may well be testing a subskill involved in reading. Most, but by no means all, poor readers, in fact, perform better on the WISC Performance sub-tests than on the Verbal sub-tests, which is not surprising, of course. The problem is further compounded by the fact that dyslexic children have been found to have difficulties in handling verbal information, in memory for reversed digits, in coding information and in arithmetic as well as in word recognition. The Wechsler test includes sub-tests for Information, Arithmetic, Digit span and Coding. The BAS includes similar sub-tests and also has sub-tests of Immediate and Delayed Recall and of Word Reading. It has, therefore, been argued that the full scores from these tests underestimate the abilities of these children because they include scores on sub-tests which reflect their constitutional dyslexia or reading difficulties. This could have the effect of so depressing a child's level of ability, as measured by the tests, that he might be considered of below average ability which, in turn, might be regarded as accounting for his reading difficulties. This is not special pleading but a problem inherent in using the tests.

Administering the tests is one thing, interpreting the results is another. But, taken in relation to all the other data about the children, the tests provide valuable indicators of children's cognitive abilities which are involved in learning generally and contribute to building up a profile of their strengths and weaknesses. The fact that the tests reflect both reasons for the children's difficulties and the results of those difficulties serves to show that the children have difficulties. Whether or not the scores should be enhanced or pro-rated to allow for scores on sub-tests in which some dyslexic or severely reading retarded pupils score badly is of academic interest. What is disappointing is that, so far, no one has been able to diagnose dyslexia or reading difficulties from these tests alone and the best that can be said of them in this respect is that their interpretation may reveal some contributory or corroborative factors and provide pointers to the strengths which may be used to help children overcome their weaknesses.

Reading Tests

Tests of reading abound. One investigator identified over seventy reading skills which various tests attempt to assess from letter recognition to speed of comprehension. But there is no test which distinguishes between dyslexic children and retarded readers. Word recognition and sentence completion tests, which are commonly used in schools and in surveys of reading ability, are crude measures which enable children to be sorted out in some sort of order according to the levels of reading ability sampled by the tests. Taken on their own, the results of these tests tell us very little about an individual child and may be misleading. A child aged 9 years with a Reading Age of 9 years on a word-recognition test appears to be reading satisfactorily but if we also know that she has difficulty in understanding reading books at that level of difficulty and has the abilities of an 11-year-old, as evidenced by her attainment on the WISC test, we will place less reliance on the significance of the Reading Age and consider her to be performing below her ability.

Although many of these tests have been standardized and correlated with one another, so that it is possible to adjust scores on one test to conform with scores on another, this does not mean that an individual child will get the same score or reading age, after the adjustments have been made, on another of the tests. On average the adjustments are useful enough but individual performance varies considerably. The child who scored satisfactorily on the word-recognition test may well have scored much lower on a sentence-completion test if she has comprehension difficulties; alternatively she may well have scored much higher if she is skilled in using contextual cues. Recently, for research purposes, we used four different tests to measure the reading ability of dyslexic and reading retarded pupils. Each child performed differently on the different tests, used different strategies on the tests and none of the tests distinguished between dyslexic and retarded pupils. But each test told us that the children had reading difficulties — which is what we knew already. A psychologist may well use such tests when he doesn't already know how a child is performing in reading but he will place more reliance on a sentence-completion test than upon a word-recognition test, will interpret the results in relation to all the other data he has, and be well aware that the test has many limitations. As we have indicated elsewhere, such tests have very limited value. An educational psychologist is much more likely to use a diagnostic reading test.

Diagnosing reading difficulties

As reading is the decoding and understanding of language it might be thought that tests of the various skills and subskills involved in the process would be available which enable the diagnostician to identify in which part or parts of the process a child was failing, having difficulty or succeeding. So far it has to be said that no such test has been developed which is better than carefully and perceptively attending to what the child does in attempting to read. The best tests simply make that possible by providing texts of graded difficulty. Attempts to go beyond this and break the skills down to enable us to predict which children will have difficulties or to identify components of the skills, such as memory for shapes or the ability to match shapes, rarely succeed in providing any more information than is available by direct observation, by using the sub-tests in the ability tests such as the Wechsler (WISC), or by using tests which are specifically designed to test discrete skills or abilities such as auditory or visual perception. Even when such tests succeed in testing only what they purport to test, which is by no means easy, it does not follow that performance on a test necessarily indicates how a child will perform in reading. As we have seen, cross-lateral children, with mixed hand, ear, eye and foot co-ordination, frequently have no reading difficulties. In the following sections we comment on a few of the more commonly used tests in the diagnosis of reading difficulties.

One of the most important functions anyone looking closely at children with reading difficulties can perform is to examine the children's language development. A number of tests are available which contribute to this investigation but, in those cases in which a detailed analysis is thought necessary, the Language Assessment, Remediation and Screening Procedure (LARSP) developed by Crystal, Fletcher and Garman, is indispensable. Against the stages of normal grammatical, or syntactical, development the user can identify abnormal or uneven development in the child's actual use of language and then prescribe the appropriate remedial measure.

The Illinois Test of Psycholinguistic Abilities (ITPA), based on Osgood's model of learning and language acquistion, although widely used, has been criticized both in its basic conception and because doubts have been expressed about the ability of its various sub-tests to have sufficiently predictive or diagnostic value. The test consists of twelve sub-tests: auditory and visual reception, visual and auditory sequential memory, auditory and visual association, visual, auditory and grammatic closure, manual and verbal expression and sound blending. Its comprehensiveness, and the inclusion of subskills with which some children have difficulty, has made it attractive to remedial teachers and many remedial programmes have been developed upon its model. Certainly the sub-tests do not distinguish discretely enough between the sensory channels they attempt to test and many psychologists consider the ITPA provides them with no information they cannot more readily and more accurately derive from tests such as WISC or BAS.

Although The Standard Reading Tests (Daniels and Diack) provides a ready means of checking reading attainment and diagnosing some of the difficulties experienced by children, particularly in the early stages of learning to read, it is not sufficiently discriminating when used with children with severe and complex difficulties. As a classroom tool, however, which is the purpose for which it was designed, it is easy to use, while in a clinical situation it can provide a quick way of establishing that more obvious deficiencies have not been overlooked.

The Neale Analysis of Reading Abilities, however, remains the most widely used and most useful test the psychologist has for diagnosing difficulties. This is an individual and on-task test in which the child reads paragraphs of graded difficulty. Besides providing assessments of accuracy, comprehension and rate of reading, the test also includes diagnostic tests from which the tester can identify mispronunciations, substitutions, refusals, additions, omissions and reversals. The test is standardized on norms for the 6–13 year age group but can be used with older retarded readers. By attending closely to the child's responses and recording them, a useful amount of information can be gathered for subsequent analysis. In our own research the responses of the dyslexic and severely reading retarded pupils were tape-recorded to minimize the possibility of missing or misinterpreting them. While the analyses of errors clearly identified individual strengths and weaknesses, we were unable, however, to distinguish between dyslexic and severely reading retarded children on the basis of the kinds of errors or the frequency with which they occurred. In other words we were unable to find one common error or common group of errors which was made only by the dyslexic pupils. When, however, the test is used to determine, for the purposes of multidisciplinary assessment, whether or not the children have a reading difficulty, the Neale Test proves perfectly adequate as an indicator of the degree of retardation if results are compared with children's performance and ability on such tests as the WISC.

The question now confronting a psychologist who has decided that there is a marked disparity between a child's general ability and his or her reading is, "Has the child a significantly greater difficulty in learning than the majority of children?" He may well consider that the reading difficulties can be accounted for by poor teaching and can be overcome by remedial teaching in the child's school or that other factors he has noted may account for the reading difficulties. Even the degree of disparity between the results of reading tests and ability tests is not, in itself, evidence of constitutional disabilities, as in the case of Frank who at twelve had a reading age of 6 years and was of average ability but, as a member of a travelling family, had rarely attended school for more than two or three weeks at a time. In the absence of any factors to account for the reading difficulties the psychologist may well decide to investigate the visual perceptual or perceptual-motor development of children.

Assessing perceptual development

The two most commonly used tests are the Marianne Frostig Test of

Visual Perception and the various forms of the Bender-Gestalt Test. The Frostig Test investigates hand–eye co-ordination, figure–ground discrimination (the ability to distinguish a shape from its background), form constancy, spatial orientation and spatial relationships. This has not proved to be a particularly discriminating or predictive instrument when used in connection with reading difficulties. When administered by someone trained in its use it is of value with children who have marked co-ordination problems, however, and the associated perceptual training programme helps these children in hand–eye co-ordination and in the development of perceptual abilities. It is rare that difficulties of this degree of severity are encountered in children with reading difficulties and there is little evidence to justify the use of the training programme to help them. They may well make progress in performance on the programme but the problem remains of translating those skills into reading skills. Some remedial teachers have done this successfully but too many assume that the successful completion of the programme will result in an improvement in reading. This is rarely the case.

The Bender-Gestalt Test examines the perceptual and visual–motor development of children by requiring them to copy a number of two-dimensional shapes of increasing complexity. In addition to providing a measure of perceptual development, it can, in the hands of someone experienced in its use, give indicators of developmental disturbance, personality disorders, emotional problems, mental retardation, aphasic (language) disorders and brain damage. This test is easy to administer but demands careful and sensitive analysis. Where the results are abnormal they serve to alert the psychologist to the need for further investigation of the child by a paediatrician, psychiatrist or neurologist. When used with children with reading problems it also provides the opportunity to diagnose difficulties of directionality, rotation, reversal and spatial orientation. The test is constructed so that all the shapes should normally be reproduced by eleven-year-olds. Although aspects of visual–motor and visual–spatial development are investigated in the Block Design Subtest of the WISC, many psychologists consider the use of the Bender-Gestalt test, in one or other of its forms, useful in any detailed investigation of children's psychological difficulties. In attempts to diagnose dyslexia the test may well indicate delayed development and visual perceptual difficulties and as a maturational lag is often said to underlie dyslexic pupils' problems, the use of the test in investigating reading difficulties is common. However, research evidence casts serious doubt on both the predictive and diagnostic value of the test and, while it may help to illuminate some aspects of children's reading difficulties, caution must be exercised in drawing conclusions from it.

In this situation, therefore, it might be thought that psychologists could identify dyslexia by recourse to check-lists of those symptoms or groups of symptoms, syndromes, which are considered to be associated with dyslexia. A number of such check-lists have been devised.

Check-lists of symptoms

It is not uncommon in medicine and psychological medicine for a disease or disability to have no one specific and unique symptom but a range of symptoms only one or some of which may be present in a particular patient at a particular time. It is rare, however, for the variety to be very great and for the investigator not to be able to make further tests to confirm or reject his diagnosis. As we have seen, it is because of the lack of specificity and predictiveness of the various symptoms or "soft" signs of dyslexia that doctors do not consider they are in a position to diagnose it. Psychologists are faced with precisely the same difficulty. The link between the symptoms and the reading difficulties is tenuous and the evidence tentative or equivocal.

A number of the factors will already have been investigated by the psychologist in his collection of data about the child. He will have discussed the circumstances surrounding the child's birth with the parents and be in a position to determine whether or not perinatal factors may have some significant bearing on the child's difficulties. He may well have investigated lateral dominance, perhaps using the Harris Tests of Lateral Dominance. The various sub-tests of the WISC will have identified children who have difficulties with information processing or coding, etc. When he turns to the check-lists he will find that some or all of these are included. Many lists look like a list of the sub-tests in WISC, the Illinois Test of Psycholinguistics and other tests he has administered or decided not to use because of doubts he had about them. The fact that one list includes one set of symptoms and another a different set simply reflects the fact that the compilers, like the children, are different and see the problem from different standpoints.

Some lists give differential weighting to the various factors, others state them baldly. Spatial difficulties, sequencing difficulties, clumsiness, mirror writing, poor memory for visual or verbal information, failure or fatigue in tasks involving auditory and visual memory, developmental delay, reversal of letters, bizarre spelling, arithmetic difficulties and hand–eye co-ordinatory problems evidenced in handwriting difficulties, are symptoms which appear in a number of check-lists. Psychologists may consider these symptoms as providing corroborative evidence of either dyslexia, specific reading retardation or a specific learning difficulty in reading, or they may regard them as interesting factors in the profiles of the children's strengths and weaknesses and general development which have little or no bearing on their reading problems. A number of them may be considered as a result, rather than a cause, of their reading retardation, while others, psychologists may well dismiss as irrelevant, because they have assessed many children with similar profiles who were successful readers.

None of this alters the fact that the children with severe reading difficulties may well need special educational provision or some form of remedial help but, in the absence of reliable indicators of the reasons for the difficulties, psychologists are again no better placed than doctors or anyone else to discriminate between dyslexic and reading retarded pupils. What will influence them most in any diagnosis they make is their assessment of the degree of retardation. Whatever their own conceptualization of dyslexia and the weight they give to its symptoms, the one piece of unequivocal evidence they may have is that a child is clearly retarded in reading. To satisfy themselves on this point, they are at pains to make allowance for the fact that there is no one-to-one correlation between tests of intelligence or ability and tests of reading. But, having made whatever adjustments are necessary for the low correlation between the ability and reading tests, established that not only is there a disparity between a child's general level of ability and his or her reading ability, and that they have so far identified no environmental or constitutional factors to account for it, psychologists may decide to look more closely at other dimensions of the child. And many psychologists will investigate more intensively even where no marked disparity between reading ability and general ability exists if children are experiencing difficulties in learning to read.

Other dimensions of difficulties

So far we have concentrated upon those aspects of dyslexia which have preoccupied researchers. Diverse though they appear at first sight they are in fact exclusively concerned with cognitive aspects or with neurological and sensory factors which affect learning. While this may be justified on the grounds of the demands of research design which, as we have seen, proceeds by a process of exclusion of those factors which might have caused reading difficulties such as sensory defects or emotional problems, it cannot be justified when we are assessing an individual child. If assessment is first of all the systematic collection of information about a child, then we need as much information as we can get or we may well ignore vital dimensions of the child of far greater significance than a difficulty in reading.

One dimension is that of the cumulative effects of failure which is certainly manifest in the majority of these children. In Henry's case, for example, although he was referred for assessment because of his reading difficulties it would have been more appropriate for him to have been referred much earlier for his emotional and behavioural problems. He avoided eye contact, nibbled at his nails, kicked his feet against his chair and responded in monosyllables. It soon transpired that at 8 yrs 7 mths he was bed-wetting, was very much an isolate, and resisted going to school where he was withdrawn and backward in all subjects except mathematics and art. But Henry's test results showed that he was well above average ability. His assessment by his teacher on the Bristol Social Adjustment Guides underlined the unforthcomingness and inconsequence which were characteristic of his behaviour. But in Henry's case his maladjustment and his reading difficulties were all eventually traced back to the fact that he had started school late because of a broken leg and in the first two years of schooling he had been frequently absent with a succession of colds, mumps, measles and other children's ailments. Henry had hated his teacher and his teacher had told him and his parents that Henry was "a mess". Confused, and behind the other children for two years, Henry had seen himself as a mess and still saw himself as a mess. Being a mess, in fact, was the one thing he had successfully learned to be. What Henry needed to learn was not how to read but how to start building a better construct or perception of himself. Only then would it be possible to get near enough to Henry to help him to learn to read.

But, even with children who exhibit no overt signs of emotional or behavioural problems, it is unlikely that we can assume that intelligent children who have known years of failure have not made a variety of adjustments in order to live with themselves and others. They may well have learned a repertoire of avoidance techniques to conceal their difficulties. Some may hide behind the label of dyslexia or behind the fact that everyone knows they have reading difficulties. They are like the alcoholic who, when admonished for social drinking by his counsellor, replied: "But what do you expect? You know I'm an alcoholic!" Emotional and behavioural factors have a bearing upon the motivation of children which is itself an essential component of learning. As we discussed in connection with the reading process, the motivation to attend and the arousal of the faculties involved in reading are essential prerequisites of learning. These aspects, largely ignored in the literature, need to be examined in any assessment of these children.

Although the various tests have given some indication of how effectively children think, none we have so far discussed have examined *how* they think, how they tackle problems or the strategies they use deductively or inferentially. The psychologist may well have observed some pointers to these dimensions of the child but his training and experience enable him to go much deeper. He may well learn far more of relevance to the child's difficulties by taking the opportunity to determine whether the child thinks impulsively or reflectively and how the child has developed in the ability to form and use concepts.

Any adequate assessment of a child's learning difficulties demands that the psychologist makes a comprehensive examination of the child's personality and of his perception of himself and of others. This assessment has to be set against all the other data concerning the child's situation in the family, his relationships with parents and siblings, in the school and in the community of peers and others. It is only in this context that it is likely, except in the most obvious cases, that anything meaningful and significant can be said about the learning and reading difficulties of these children. The bland assumption that reading tests and ability tests take us very far results in the frequently uttered cry of teachers when they read reports which do little more than quote and discuss the pupils' performance on these tests: "I knew all that — that's why I wanted him examined!" Psychological assessment which is comprehensive, which includes careful and sensitive interpretation of data, and provides positive recommendations of the changes which will most effectively produce improvements in pupils' performance and well-being, is essential. The limited perspectives provided by check-lists and which look at reading and ability in isolation are largely a waste of time and only serve to confirm what was already known. Certainly that confirmation may be reassuring and trigger action, but the action that is triggered may well be completely inappropriate. Fortunately, such is the resilience of children and so pervasive the effects of success, that getting something going which does produce results may outweigh the dangers of this. In other cases, however, the action may exacerbate the underlying difficulties and the children start by not attending to the teacher and soon stop attending altogether.

If we assume that a psychological assessment has proceeded to the point at which all the dimensions of the child which we have discussed have been examined, is there anything else a psychologist may consider appropriate to diagnose dyslexia? One instrument we have not discussed is the Aston Index.

The Aston Index

The Aston Index is a battery of tests devised and validated at the Language Development Research Unit at the University of Aston, Birmingham. It is designed as a screening and diagnostic test for use by teachers, psychologists and doctors and may be used with children in the 5–14 year age-group. Level I of the Index is for use with children in the first year of school; Level II is for the diagnosis of difficulties in pupils aged 7 years and over. Diagnosis having

been made, the Index also indicates appropriate remedial programmes. The battery of sub-tests measure general ability,
vocabulary, reading, spelling, directionality, visual and auditory
sequential memory, letter sounding and blending, written expression and grapho-motor ability. As can be seen the Index tests
the same range of abilities and skills a psychologist will have
examined but has the advantage of placing in the hands of teachers
a fairly comprehensive means of making assessment and of pre-
scribing treatment. Unfortunately, perhaps in order to achieve the
latter objective, many of the tests used are those commonly used by
teachers. The reading test is a word-recognition test and is suitable
only for coarse screening, and there is no diagnostic test of reading.
The sequential memory test, while providing a means by which
teachers may test these abilities, are similar to those which a
psychologist uses in administering the WISC or BAS test. As we
have seen, sequential memory difficulties are frequently held to be
a symptom of dyslexia but the evidence for this is equivocal.
However, the Index has been widely used and there is an
abundance of supportive research literature which includes both
case-studies and statistical evidence of its validity.

We would certainly deplore the use of the Index for screening
purposes in the early years of schooling on the grounds that it
might well result in teachers lowering their expectations of children
and result in early labelling and a self-fulfilling prophecy. Rather
than waste time testing, teachers would be better employed
teaching in these early years. Certainly they have no reason to use
letter recognition tests which can only tell them a lot less than they
should know about their children's oral, reading and other
accomplishments. The Index also directs teachers' attention away
from the task of reading and into subskills and the fragmentation of
the process rather than its synthesis. Getting it all together is what
reading is all about for beginning readers.

A similar objection can be made to the use of the Index with older
children who at Level II are assessed by the word-recognition
reading test, spelling test, free-writing test and test of grapho-
motor ability. A psychologist meeting a child for the first time
might well have recourse to similar tests but a teacher working with
and observing children in the classroom should not need them and
has available, in any case, more sophisticated, more recent and
discriminating tests. The use of the Index, moreover, will again

result in teachers directing their efforts into teaching subskills. There is no doubt that these old methods do work with many teachers and children and, in so far as they work, they are not to be decried. But almost any method will work and even the absence of method, as in the case of look-and-say, will work for many children. It is disappointing to find that teachers and specialists in dyslexia so often have such a limited conceptualization of the reading process and of children's development and learning that the methods of instruction they adopt appear more appropriate to the 1880s than the 1980s.

Making a decision

Although psychologists may have difficulty in deciding whether or not children are dyslexic, they will have less difficulty in deciding whether or not the children are severely retarded in reading. They must also decide which factors appear to be militating against the children's progress and it will be rare that they will identify only one. Almost invariably there will be a concatenation of interrelated factors. These they must take into account in making recommendations as to how the special educational needs of the children are to be met. The more comprehensive their assessments have been, the better able they will be to make a judgment which encompasses the physical, educational, emotional, social and other needs of the children. One child may need motivating, another need help with emotional or behavioural difficulties, another speech therapy to develop language abilities, another the security of a small group and another the reduction of stress and anxiety. The fact that they also need help with their reading, writing and spelling may be a primary or secondary need. Until other difficulties have been alleviated, attempts to improve reading, particularly by a frontal assault from a battery of subskills, in some cases would prove counter-productive. In other cases, the need for corrective or remedial education in reading and its associated skills may be all that is needed. Whatever the case, one of the recommendations they will have to make must be the ways by which the children's reading can be improved.

Here, again, the decisions may be subject to constraints. Resources in the area may well be limited or already fully used.

Some they may consider inappropriate. They may be reluctant to send young children to special classes or units consisting of much older pupils or vice versa. Often making the right match between pupils and teachers is more important than matching children with methods. One constraint will be the psychologists' views on remediation in reading generally and on the assessments they make of the efficacy of the various teachers, remedial teachers, classes, units and clinics available. Here we can only address ourselves to the methods of remediation used with dyslexic and severely reading retarded pupils and attempt to assess them.

Remedies: types of remediation programmes

The methodology of remedial approaches to reading reflect both basic methods of teaching reading and the concepts of dyslexia or reading difficulties. The majority of approaches, so far as dyslexia is concerned, in both the USA and UK, start with the letters and their sounds, and sequence methodically to blends and digraphs of increasing complexity. Usually they attach great importance to improving auditory and visual sequencing. Many include some form of multisensory training. The teaching of letters, their shape and sound usually goes hand in hand with the teaching of writing and spelling. All this reflects the view that dyslexic children's difficulties lie in matching sounds to the printed letters and that they have some form of memory deficit.

The multisensory methods are based on the pioneer work of Edith Norrie in Denmark and Grace Fernald in the USA. They may be summed up in the phrase, "Hear it, say it, see it, write it". Fernald particularly emphasizes the use of the tactile sense, recommending that some children are helped by tracing the shape of letters on sandpaper shapes or by feeling teacher's finger making the shape on their backs as they write it in chalk on a board. These multisensory or kinaesthetic methods have been fairly widely used in remedial reading for over a quarter of a century and have been found successful because they use strong sensory channels to complement and supplement the input on the visual or auditory channels which may be defective.

In America Gillingham and Stillman, and in the UK Hornsby and Hickey, have contributed to the progressive refinement and

development of the phonic structured approaches which incor-
porate multisensory techniques. Cotterill, in particular, emphasizes the importance of a writing approach to reading as an integral
part of a structured approach.

In the Orton Society in America, the Word Blind Centre and
British Dyslexia Association in the UK, and in many clinics such as
those of the Scottish Rite Hospital, Dallas, Texas, or of the University College of North Wales, Bangor, methods similar to these
described above are advocated. The remedial programmes are
characterized, too, by careful matching to the individual child's
needs, one-to-one instruction, the reduction of anxiety and stress
and the precision of the structured programmes in which the
teacher follows the pattern: Teach, Learn, Test, Revise.

The various centres, associations and clinics have not only
helped thousands of children but, through their publications, con-
ferences and courses, they have informed the public and contributed to the education of hundreds of teachers. Increasingly
there has been a recognition of the diversity and degrees of dyslexia
and, in many instances, of the need for flexibility.

When considering placement of a child for whom a psychologist
has made a diagnosis of dyslexia or specific learning difficulty in
reading, writing and spelling, it may well be that consideration
may be given to the child attending a centre or clinic in which
approaches such as those described above are followed. In many
areas, remedial classes and centres are staffed by teachers some of
whom have been trained in the methods described and who use
materials and resources associated with the programmes. Many
parents who live remote from the major centres, clinics and
hospitals and are keen that their children should be taught in this
way should not be dismayed. In England and Wales, for instance
they must be consulted and given an opportunity to express their
wishes, as part of the procedure of making a statement about
children's special educational needs, under the Education Act,
1981. They owe it to themselves and their children, therefore, to
visit reading and remedial centres in their area and see for themselves what methods and approaches are used and make their own
assessment of how appropriate they may be to the children's
needs.

However, many classes, units and centres established by LEAs
employ a variety of approaches which differ in both theory and

practice from those associated with word-blind and dyslexia associations and clinics. Parents and psychologists alike have to determine whether the methods they use and the results they obtain are likely to meet the children's needs. The fact that dyslexic or severely retarded readers have not previously responded to remedial education is often taken by parents to mean that all school-based and local education authority remedial centres are unable to meet their children's needs and that only specialist dyslexic centres or clinics can do this. Usually, however, the remedial education the children have previously experienced in their schools may have amounted to little more than withdrawal from their classes for some individual or group reading. Increasingly, the tendency has been for classes and centres to be established staffed by specially trained teachers often working directly with the School Psychological Service or an adviser in special or remedial education. In London and Staffordshire, for example, this has been the case for decades. In many areas, but by no means all, the service provided is highly professional and caters for a whole range of reading difficulties, from those caused by cultural deprivation to severe communication difficulties. Whether or not the psychologist is directly involved with these services, he will have a close working relationship with them and is well placed to identify the most suitable class or unit if there is one.

As we have seen, moreover, while dyslexic centres and clinics have built up over the years considerable experience in helping these children, there is nothing unique in the methods they employ. Basically, they adopt a phonic and structured approach to instruction which is well understood by many experienced and specially trained teachers in local authority units. Many of the teachers, too, have a wide range of skills and expertise, backed up by resources of special aids and materials, and are accustomed to working closely with psychologists and therapists in the design and development of individual programmes. In this respect their approach may differ considerably from the approach of the dyslexic clinic. Instead of modifying one specific programme to the individual child they will select from a wide range of programmes the one considered most suitable and then tailor that to the child.

A practical example of what can be done is provided by Edwards in *Reading Problems: Identification and Treatment*. Based on work carried out in Australia, where it was first published, and subsequently revised and extended for publication in the UK, Edwards' approach is frankly eclectic. Each reading difficulty is identified, its possible causes, signs, remediation, sample exercises, teaching strategies, activities and instructional materials both commercial and teacher or pupil made, are clearly set out. Visual and auditory analysis skills, inadequate sight vocabulary and comprehension skills, the inability to use context clues and inefficient rates of reading are comprehensively examined in a thoroughly practical and workmanlike manner. It will be noted that a number of the problems dealt with are those associated with dyslexia, but what characterizes Edwards' suggested treatments is that a wide range of game-playing activities are recommended, together with alternative approaches, which sequence to on-task exercise in reading.

A simple and very effective way of relating research to helping children in the actual task of reading was demonstrated to us by Dr Matějček in Prague, Czechoslovakia. Because many of the children are found to have difficulty in focusing on or giving selective attention to the syllables of words, a piece of white card from which windows have been cut is used. The windows are just big enough for one or more letters to be exposed while the rest of the text is masked by the card. Slots of various length are also cut in the sides of the card so that the beginnings and endings of word can be isolated. When teachers use a simple device such as this, as soon as the children begin to experience difficulty, many find that this is all that is necessary to help the children scan efficiently and identify the component parts of words as sound–sense units. Placing the card just below the line being read, and quickly isolating and saying the sound or syllable over which a child hesitates, helps the child to carry on reading without any loss of the sense of the passage. On-task instruction such as this proceeds by the reduction of uncertainty and maintains the child's access to meaning.

Frequently, considerable attention is given to counselling children and their parents in order to overcome the sense of failure and anxiety and to developing positive attitudes and the children's self-esteem. Programmes may well use audio-visual aids as a means of developing the children's focus of attention and to provide both maximum impact and reinforcement. Multi-sensory approaches developed from Grace Fernald's work are commonly used and subskills of reading, writing and spelling, rather than being the main ingredient, are frequently introduced as and when children are ready to extend their repertoire of strategies. In many remedial centres the range of programmes and resources is such that they provide an approach similar to that described in Chapter 3 which enable each child to be taken through the MODES of reading by the most expeditious route to mastery.

One of the big advantages of some local authority centres and clinics is that they work closely with the schools. The aim of remediation is to get the children, wherever possible, back into the mainstream of education. If this is to be done it is essential that the programmes are designed to this end and that the children's skills in reading, writing and spelling have been developed to the point at which they can read the textbooks in ordinary schools across the curriculum, and are able to write up their assignments, projects, notes and homework. It is not enough that they have merely reached their chronological age on a word-recognition test which provides no measure of their ability to cope with mainstream education: they must be functionally literate in the educational environment appropriate to their age and ability. Clearly, working with specialist teachers familiar with the schools is the best guarantee that this will be done. Once returned to their schools, their progress will continue to be monitored and, should the need arise, additional support and help can be provided. These remedial centres have a vested interest in ensuring that the needs of the children, their parents and the schools are all being met.

Beyond remediation

Multidisciplinary assessment and the remediation of reading difficulties, no matter how thorough and effective it may be, is picking up the pieces and making the best of a bad job. Why should we wait until children are failing? If remedial methods, which contain no magic ingredients, produce results, why weren't the methods a part of ordinary teaching? If the instruments of assessment are so crude and suspect, why should we use them at all? If we accept, as accept we must, that some children have severe difficulties in learning to read, which may remain with them all their lives, why don't we accept the responsibility for identifying and providing for them in our schools from the start? If we value literacy in our society, why don't we deliver it in a way which meets the needs of all our children and young people? Why do we make stopgap and *ad hoc* provision for those who we know are trapped in the cycle of cultural deprivation, have emotional problems, are below average ability or have constitutional reading difficulties?

The value and the effectiveness of remedial reading has frequently been questioned. Its value has been challenged not only because in many cases the need for it could have been avoided but also because it usually treats reading as an isolated skill rather than in the context of the children's education. Its effectiveness is also difficult to substantiate. Frequently children make initial gains in reading which, a year later, are found not to have been sustained. The most positive evidence suggests that it is only when pupils have been helped to make considerable improvement in both their skills and their attitudes to reading that the likelihood of them again falling back is reduced.

The evidence also points to the importance of the early identification of difficulties and their speedy correction; the longer the problems persist, the more complex and intractable they become and the more difficult and protracted their remediation. It is in this context that we need a new perspective on the education of dyslexic or severely reading retarded children. The problems of defining their difficulties, of diagnosing and remediating them, alerts us to the inadequacy of our understanding of the diversity of children in our schools and of people in our society, and to the poverty of our understanding of how we teach reading.

As Ruth Strang urged many years ago, we need to have clear goals or objectives for the teaching of reading, writing and spelling and, "by bridging the existing gap between practice and psychological theory and research", develop ways by which we "may prevent much childhood failure and discouragement". We believe that there is now sufficient theory, research and examples of good practice which point to how this can be done.

CHAPTER 7

The Problem in Perspective

"Human beings don't grasp what isn't fiercely
expressed." Saul Bellow

The interest and controversy aroused by the parents of dyslexic children and public concern about standards of literacy have focused attention upon the need for more research into a process we take almost for granted as a natural human attribute. There has been, too, a demand for more effective measures to identify and meet the needs of children as early as possible. But at national and local levels, some parents are still unconvinced that those responsible for the administration of education have the will, expertise and resources to help their children, and are driven to seek help in the clinics and units they are helping to finance through their voluntary efforts.

In this last respect the position of these parents *vis à vis* the educational system differs from that of parents of children with other handicaps. All that parents of dyslexic or severely reading retarded children are asking is that their children should be taught to read, that they be given the very skill of literacy which our educational systems were established to provide. The setting up of remedial centres, adult literacy or Headstart projects, is only a partial response to a deeper and more extensive social problem. Something more fundamental and effective is demanded.

The Need for Change

It is easy enough to say that the demands and the need for literacy in the Third World require the incentives, opportunities and resources to enable the people to learn to read. In the developed world, where we have the incentives, opportunities and resources, we must ask ourselves why we are still failing so many. Perhaps the answer lies in the fact that we have become so institutionalized that we are failing to harness the expertise, resources and energies we have. Cipolla, in his *Literacy and Development in the West* (1969), puts the problem in that context:

> An advanced industrial society will be characterised, at least for some time to come, by a high degree of technological change. Under this condition, the best solutions are those which inherently contain *a high degree of flexibility and adaptability to change.*
>
> In a highly dynamic industrial environment, an educational institution, no matter how excellent, is bound to become rapidly obsolete if it is hampered by traditionalism and if its change is dependent upon complicated and time-consuming bureaucratic procedures. Ultimately the effectiveness of an institution depends upon the quality of its members and of their leaders, but there is no doubt that rigid institutional arrangements can frustrate and obliterate *a generous amount of goodwill and human energy.* (Our italics.)

If we are to find the best solutions which contain a high degree of flexibility and adaptability to change and harness a generous amount of goodwill and human energy, then certain facts need to be clearly stated. First, we must recognize the need for increasingly higher levels of literacy. Both the quality and rapidity of social, cultural and technological change demand this. Second, we must recognize that our concern for higher levels of literacy must be given a central place in our concern for education generally. It cannot be separated off as an isolated skill with sub-sets of subskills and higher order skills taught by specialists. Reading in our society is central to the development of thought and language and to the educational process. Its aims and objectives must be clearly established. If this is to be done then it is vital that we recognize, with Jerome Bruner, that like everything else we wish to communicate to our children, "a theory of development must be linked both to a theory of knowledge and to a theory of instruction, or be doomed to triviality". Finally, we must be as concerned for reading to be taught in such a way that it meets the needs of all children, whether they have constitutional difficulties, defects, disabilities or handicaps, emotional or behavioural problems, lower than average levels of general ability or suffer from social and cultural deprivation.

The needs of dyslexic pupils can no longer be narrowly conceived by exclusionary definitions hedged round by obfuscating qualifications and circular arguments. They have difficulties in learning to read and they will be best helped if they are taught early enough and well enough in a way which teaches them to learn to read by reading. Labelling them and isolating them can only result in divisive, piecemeal and partial measures, in the ill-effects of a self-fulfilling prophecy and in lower expectations. "Dyslexic" will become another playground taunt just like the labels moron, cretin, dumb and spastic. They have a clear "right to read" which they share with all children whatever their difficulties or special educational, social or other needs.

For many years we have been insisting that only a holistic theory of reading could provide an adequate base from which to advance. Almost invariably, however, the response has been that that was all very well for the generality of children but it did not meet the needs of slow learners, retarded readers or dyslexic pupils. For them only a diet of phonics and subskills was appropriate. A similar response greeted Frank Smith's insistence that it is only through reading that children learn to read. But it is only in recent years that the evidence has been building up to demonstrate that the theory and instructional methods derived from it work for all children.

Marie Clay, in New Zealand, summed up the position when she wrote:

All understandings of how we read, and of what the reading process is, have changed in the last fifteen years under the impact of reports from intensive research efforts. What the old scholars recommend as techniques still have validity; the ways in which they understood the reading process do not. Theorists now look upon the reading process in a different way and that makes many of the older books on reading out of date. It is not enough today to recommend old concepts and cures to solve reading difficulties. We now have very good reasons for discarding old concepts that led to ineffective teaching.

'Reading Recovery' in New Zealand

It was from this base that, in 1976, when Marie Clay headed the "Reading Recovery" Research in Auckland, that she discerned that good readers ask themselves effective questions for reducing uncertainty while poor readers ask trivial questions. And many remedial programmes direct their students to the trivial questions. All readers, from the 5-year-old on his first book, to the efficient adult use

- the sense
- the sentence structure
- order
- size
- special features
- special knowledge
- the first and last letter cues

before they resort to left to right sounding of letters. This is what makes the terms "look and say", "sight words" and "phonics" nonsense as explanations of what we do when we read, and what we need to do in order to be able to read.

When she designed her three-year research programme to identify and help 6-year-olds who were failing in reading, she posed the question: "Can we use the collective experience of good teachers to develop and describe some teaching procedures that can be used with failing children?" The results of her research with pupils with a variety of reading, language and cultural difficulties demonstrates the power of the model of reading she used. The children's difficulties were diagnosed not by tests but by close observation of what they were saying and doing in reading; by observing what they could do rather than what they couldn't do; by discovering what they could learn next in reading rather than in puzzles and kits; and by shifting the children's reading behaviours from the less adequate to the more adequate rather than in visual or auditory perceptual training programmes. Teaching was based on the principles of individual, intensive and consistent tuition. Children were not classified or categorized but programmes were developed, meticulously monitored and assessed according to how effectively they met each child's needs. Except for research purposes, the children were not tested in reading but were assessed according to the primers or basal readers they could read and by the criteria of the cues they used in reading. With very few exceptions, the children made significant progress. The whole approach to both diagnosis and remediation was 'on task' and a model of the interactive process by which teachers use their skills and their understanding of the process itself, and of the strategies used by the child, to enable the child to become self-improving in reading. The value of the Project in terms of the happiness and competence of the children who were helped to become self-improving pupils in the mainstream of education cannot be overestimated. The effectiveness and the economy of programmes such as this, which identify difficulties early and have a preventative function, have everything to commend them to parents, teachers and administrators.

But if our models of reading and of instruction are so powerful it should be possible to extend and develop them. Clay used the existing resources of teachers, books and materials in the schools. She questioned the validity of amateurs helping children with reading difficulties and stressed the importance of the teacher with specialist knowledge and an understanding of the process of reading. For our part, while in no way questioning that thoroughly professional stance, *we have long believed that there is a "generous amount of goodwill and human energy" about and that we should have the flexibility and adaptability in our literate community to harness it.*

Parents as a resource of energy and goodwill

The needs of the children and the needs of society cannot wait upon the slow processes by which ideas percolate through educational systems before they are translated into action by new generations of teachers who then discover they are out-dated and inappropriate. Nor need we wait upon retraining if new and untapped resources are at hand. In the education of children one resource which is usually available is the parents. Their role as partners in meeting the needs of children with handicaps and difficulties is now firmly established. Moreover, a number of projects, such as those in the London Borough of Haringey and in Lancashire, have demonstrated the contribution parents can make to helping their children learn to read. But, as we have already seen, not only is the interest and support of parents of vital importance if children are to derive the maximum benefit of educational provisions, one of the most important contributions parents do make is in equipping their children with language and with the beginnings of literacy. The children who come to school already beginning to read and to write, and each year thousands of them do, are off to a flying start. If learning to read is best facilitated by the sensitive interaction between the learner and someone who already understands the process on an individual basis, then who could be better than a parent who also understands the child?

It is a big jump from this proposition to our next, which is that parents of children with severe difficulties may also be able to help them. It was this hypothesis which we decided to explore in the authors' own action-research designed to try to help dyslexic children to learn to read.

Action Research for Dyslexic Pupils

The action research project which we designed had as its aim the improvement of the reading skills of fifteen children between the ages of 8 and 13 years in three counties. The project was advertised in the local press and invited the parents of children who had been diagnosed as dyslexic by recognized independent specialists or clinics to take part. From the twenty-five applications we received we selected fifteen children, twelve boys and three girls, in the age-group, all of whom were two or more years retarded in reading, had regularly attended school and had been independently diagnosed as dyslexic. We then asked schools similar to those attended by these pupils to provide us with the names of any of their pupils who were severely retarded in reading. There was no shortage of such pupils and we tested a group of about 300 pupils in the 8–13 age-group.

From this group, as accurately as possible, thirty pupils were selected who matched the dyslexic pupils in age, sex, reading level and general ability. The parents of fifteen of this matched group were invited to take part in the project, and these children became the Matched Group. The remaining fifteen pupils became the Control Group. No one else knew who was in the Control Group and they took no further part in the project until it ended when their reading was re-tested.

The parents of the fifteen pupils in the Dyslexic Group and the fifteen pupils in the Matched Group were asked to give their children 30 minutes instruction a day for a year and to allow their children to attend three Holiday Schools for a week in each of the three school holidays.

From our previous experience in working with parents, and from our observations of Portage projects in which parents are helped to contribute to the development and education of their handicapped children, we knew that it was essential to give parents clear guidelines on what to do. We also knew that they would need help and support during the year. We therefore spent a day familiarizing the parents with how we wanted them to teach their children and with the books, materials and activities they would be using. We also appointed a Teacher-Researcher who would visit them regularly in their homes and act as a professional guide, comforter and friend. The parents were asked to start the day after their induction session.

The project ran for a year, at the end of which we re-tested the reading of all the thirty children in the Dyslexic and Matched Groups and of the fifteen children in the Control Group. The results for the three Groups of children are shown in Fig. 7, p. 144. As can be seen, all the children who had been helped by their parents were markedly superior in their reading abilities, as measured by the test, to the children in the Control Group. Only two children in the Control Group had made more than a year's progress in the year; one child in the group actually scored less than he had done at the beginning of the year. In other words, with two exceptions, all the children in the Control Group were further behind in reading than they had been so far as their test results were concerned.

Figure 7 Gains in reading made by the experimental and control groups in one year

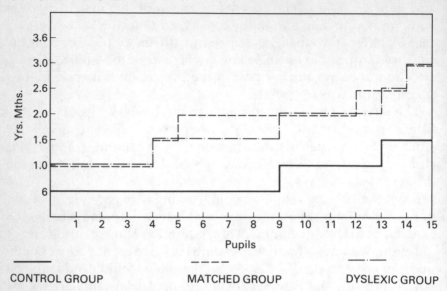

CONTROL GROUP   MATCHED GROUP   DYSLEXIC GROUP

As the ceiling or maximum age measured by the Test was 10 yrs 6 mths, the full extent of the gains made by some pupils, who scored the maximum "reading age", in the Experimental Groups, are not shown here.

The Real Results

The results also showed that there was virtually no difference between the reading levels of the Dyslexic and the Matched Groups. Whatever had been done had proved to be equally appropriate to the needs of the two groups of children. The progress made by these children, moreover, was statistically significant. One pupil had made 4 years' progress, ten had made 3–4 years' progress and eleven had made 2–3 years' progress. Educationally, however, their progress was even more impressive. Although, for the purposes of the research, we had used a variety of reading tests in parallel versions, we had monitored the children's progress both on the books they were able to read and in the changes in their reading behaviours. We did this by direct observation of the pupils during the Holiday Schools; by recording the information collected by the Teacher Researcher; and by asking the parents and the children. By the end of the year ten of the children were able to read and understand adult texts. Parents and pupils independently reported an overall, and in some cases dramatic, improvement in school work. Books were being read for pleasure in bed or in free time. Books were being read for information in connection with hobbies, homework and school projects. Newspapers, magazines and comics were now widely read. The majority of parents, and of children themselves, considered that they were adequate or good readers. Spelling had improved and many children were now expressing themselves efficiently and fluently in writing for the first time. All the parents reported that relations with their children had improved or remained good throughout the year.

When we had designed this project we had hoped that it would enable us to identify ways by which other children with similar difficulties might be helped. But we had to wait until we had analysed the results at the end of the year before doing this. We also had to avoid making too many changes during the year in what the parents were doing as this would have made it even more difficult to determine what had worked and what had failed. Clearly, whatever we might learn would only be of value in so far as we realized our aim of improving the reading of the dyslexic pupils. All the research evidence pointed to the fact that we were unlikely to succeed to any significant extent in realizing this aim. Thus, when we first became aware of the progress a number of the pupils had made in the first ten weeks of the project, we attributed this to the Hawthorne effect. This effect affects all research. It was found in the Hawthorne works of the Western Electricity Company in America in 1939 that, if lighting and working conditions were improved, production improved but then tailed off; turn down the lighting and reduce the incentives, and production again improves and, again, tails off. So we allowed for this effect and waited for the children's progress to drop back. By the mid-term of the project, however, the progress was still, in many cases, accelerating and outstripping the gentle and careful rate for which we had planned. Still mindful of the research evidence, we advanced the level of the difficulty of the books for these pupils as far as we considered it safe to do. We warned the parents that the early gains might not be maintained and that, at the first sign of difficulties, we would provide less demanding books. But the difficulties never came and we had been wrong. The parents and the children, what is more, told us we had been wrong. Far more rapidly than we would have believed possible in our most euphoric moments, many of the children had progressed from being dyslexic and severely retarded readers to being print-borne and from being print-borne to book-hooked. With the benefit of hindsight, and after a closer look at the reading skills of the individual children concerned, we can only state that, had we had more confidence in what we and the parents had been doing, and in our models of reading and reading instruction, many of these pupils would have made even greater progress.

What the parents did

What produced such improvements in the children's reading which is of relevance to other parents, teachers and educational administrators? Undoubtedly, the active interest and involvement of the parents was the major factor. But how were the parents involved and what did they do?

1. At the start, the children were given books which were about two years below their levels of reading ability.
2. The parents read to and with their children and heard their children read a few pages of the books each day for not more than a total of fifteen minutes.
3. The parents used the passages the children had read as the basis for playing a variety of word games and other activities with their children each day for a maximum of fifteen minutes.
4. Included in the activities were simple substitution codes ($A = 1$, $B = 2$, etc), write-and-spell, and a collection of nonsense rhymes; these were rotated with the other activities over a period of three days to ensure variety.

No remedial methods or techniques were used and the main activities were on-task and designed to focus the children's attention upon developing strategies for using the various cues in the texts they had read. Writing and spelling went hand in hand with this. Initially, many children had to be taught how to hold their pencils, position the paper and form letters in an efficient cursive style; this was done in the context of teaching them to spell. The codes were included because coding is an activity in which dyslexic pupils are said to find difficulty. The nonsense rhymes served the purpose of developing language awareness, the memorization of verbal material, and giving the children and their parents fun. The reading books provided were selected so that, from the outset, they were well within each child's competency. So far as possible, we wanted children and parents to find it easy. Children whose reading abilities, as shown by the tests, were at the 6 or 7-year-old level, were therefore given picture books with a minimum of text and these were used largely as a means of developing conversation about the text and the pictures. However, care was taken in the selection of books to ensure that they were of interest to the children, appeared to be for children of the same age or older, and that they were not books they would have met in school. The majority of children were given the "Trend" (Ginn) series which met these criteria.

Paired-reading

Starting the children off with easy books played a major part in the success of the project. Too often in the remediation of reading teachers find the children's "reading ages" and start teaching them at just below that level. Remediation should start at the level at which the child is completely secure and can be successful. But, with children who have known years of failure, even being asked to read aloud to mother or father is a daunting and threatening experience. We wanted the experience to be enjoyable and free of stress from the outset for, we realized, if it began badly, there was a danger of both children and parents opting out.

To build success upon success, therefore, we asked the parents to follow a set procedure with the fifteen minute reading sessions. Having first read the passage, the parent then:

1. Talks about the passage, the pictures, characters, the story so far, with the child for two or three minutes.
2. Reads the passage aloud as naturally and with as much expression as possible, while running a finger along under the lines of print, for three minutes.
3. Reads the passage aloud with the child joining in, in unison, i.e. paired-reading, for three minutes.

4. Reads the passage aloud with the child in unison, but this time pausing occasionally for the child to provide the next word or phrase at points in the text where the parent is reasonably certain the child will be able to carry on; three minutes.
5. The child reads the passage aloud. Should the child hesitate the parent supplies the word or phrase; three minutes.

The parents were asked to praise the children for attending, for joining in, for reading with expression, for supplying the right word or phrase and for effort or improvement. Confrontation was to be avoided at all costs. For the majority of children the experience of being praised for their performance of a task they associated with failure was dramatic. A few weeks after the start of the project, one parent reported that her daughter Marilyn came home from school, threw down her satchel, danced through the house and out round the garden. Asked what had happened, Marilyn replied; "Nothing. I've just realized — reading's easy! You just have to make it mean sense! I'd never seen that before." Another parent commented: "If only I'd known how easy it is to help John — I could have saved us both years of misery". However, when Mark's mother first praised his reading, his response was a derisory: "You must be joking!" Wisely she adopted a more matter-of-fact attitude. When, a week or so later, Mark had done particularly well, and she said, "Not bad," Mark replied with a knowing wink.

Prepared reading

For some of the older or more able readers, paired-reading, having got the children and parents started successfully, was no longer necessary. It was replaced with "prepared reading". The Teacher-Researcher showed the parents how to first read a passage aloud and then go through it with the children, drawing attention to words and phrases the meaning or reading of which might cause difficulty. Only then were the children asked to read aloud on their own. This made absolutely sure that no child was ever asked to read anything he didn't understand. Again, the parents were encouraged to supply any words or phrases over which the children found difficulty. Prepared reading had the added advantage of allowing much more time for the children's own reading during the fifteen-minute sessions. They got more quickly into the stories and were keen to find out what happened next. They were now reading for pleasure and expressing their individual preferences for books. The Teacher-Researcher fed this interest by leaving a wide selection of books, appropriate to the children's interests and abilities, and encouraged the parents to let the children choose the books they wanted to read. Some children were soon getting book-hooked.

Activities

Parents varied considerably in their ability to match the tasks to the texts and to their children's abilities and interests. But all persevered. Surprisingly, many dyslexic pupils were fascinated with the codes. The nonsense rhymes and crossword puzzles were so successful with some children and their parents that they bought books of rhymes and codes. The write-and-spell activities enabled some children to unlearn their old inefficient habits and to start writing legibly and efficiently for the first time. Some children insisted, quite rightly, that they must conform to their schools' handwriting style and the Teacher-Researcher helped parents bridge this gap. Again, parents were advised to encourage and praise their children in their performance of these tasks and to keep them as closely related to the reading as possible.

The Holiday Schools

These were included in the project for two reasons: we wanted to be able to monitor the children's progress; we wanted to individualize the programmes and complement and supplement the work being done by the parents. We also wanted to use educational plant and resources which lie idle in holiday times. The Schools were staffed by experienced remedial teacher advisers who we trained in the use of the same methods and procedures as those being used by the parents. Reading activities were limited to four half-hour sessions per day, the rest of the time being given over to games, art-and-craft, video-films and other activities which were as enjoyable and as relaxed as we could make them for the children.

The first School was in the middle of the summer holiday. Not only did all the children attend but they surprised everyone by the speed and enthusiasm with which they settled down. The teachers all commented on their excellent work-habits. This was a remarkable tribute to the parents' success and something we had not anticipated. The children were all familiar with paired-reading, the majority read their books with confidence and knew precisely what to do and how to do the various activities. The project had only been running two months. At the end of the week the children suggested that in future Schools they would prefer forty-minute sessions of reading activities, "to get more work done"!

The second Holiday School began on the 28 December which we regarded as as big a disincentive as could be devised. One child was in hospital. Everyone else arrived from the three counties and settled straight down to work. For the first time since the project began, we re-tested the children's reading and had our first objective evidence of the progress many had made. The teachers confirmed our assessment of the cautious extent to which it was thought safe to accelerate some of the children. Again the remedial teachers eschewed their own preferred methods and co-operated by adhering to the same methods as the parents. They were particularly successful in helping some of the younger and the most retarded children and provided valuable advice which the Teacher-Researcher conveyed to the parents.

At the third and final Holiday School the twelve boys and girls, about whose substantial progress there was now no doubt, were placed in two groups and their teachers were asked to see how far the pupils could go in coping with more difficult and unprepared texts. Here we were applying a concept first described by Vygotsky in the 1930s in Russia. He described how some children reach a level of development in a cognitive ability and are perfectly able to go beyond it. Other children can go only a little way forward. Some are unable to go forward at all. Vygotsky calls this "a zone of proximal (or potential) development". For example, in mathematics, in a group of children who have just learned simple multiplication of decimals by whole numbers, some may be able to do long multiplication and division of decimal numbers, some to do multiplication and division of decimals by whole numbers, and some to multiply by decimal numbers, without further instruction. Others remain stuck at multiplying decimal numbers by whole numbers. The extent of the zone of proximal development is an indication of how well the pupils understand the particular concept and its relation to other concepts and skills they know, and their ability to apply the new concept or skill. Bruner refers to the similar ability to "go beyond the information given". We wanted to see how far the pupils could use their reading abilities because we were still unsure that they had yet reached the stage either of competency or mastery in reading. Confronted with more difficult and unseen texts we anticipated that they would become insecure and be denied access to meaning.

The teachers soon found that all these children were perfectly able to read the most difficult books in the series we had been using. They were then given textbooks in school subjects for pupils of their own age. The teachers were surprised at the confidence with which they tackled them. We were now convinced that we had not yet reached the limits of their potential. The only adequate test was to give them adult texts to read. On a shelf in the staffroom we found a row of *Readers' Digest* magazines. We gave them to the pupils and suggested they looked through them to see if there were any articles or stories that interested them. In a few minutes they were all busily reading. When we heard Marilyn reading about neurosurgery, John off on a safari with wardens keeping vigil against ivory poachers, Paul in outer space, Lennie deep into oceanography with remote-controlled bathyspheres, and Mark engrossed in erupting Icelandic volcanoes, we were convinced. They did not notice that not only were they tackling words of considerable "phonic" difficulty, they were reading and understanding compound and complex sentences in which the meaning was often deeply embedded. Their zones of proximal development extended way beyond functional literacy. In conversation with them, it was clear that they were perfectly able to relate what they had learned in school, at home or from television about the subjects about which they were reading and use this knowledge as participants in the process. Reading had become an automatized and self-rewarding, self-improving skill.

A problem with homework

As a number of the children were already in comprehensive

schools when the project started, and as their parents had assured us that what little homework a few of them had presented no difficulty as far as the half-hour's project work was concerned, we were unprepared for what happened in September. A number of these pupils were moved into new forms and a number of the 11-year-olds transferred to comprehensive schools. To their parents' delight many were placed not in remedial classes but in mainstream classes because of the progress they had made. But, to their parents' dismay, they all came home with homework in English, history, geography, science, mathematics and French. For many of these pupils the textbooks and assignments were beyond them. Parents complained to the Teacher-Researcher that they couldn't possibly continue with the project work each evening when their children had as much as two hours' homework. The Teacher-Researcher suggested that the parents should use the same methods with the homework as they had used with the project activities but advised that they should keep the reading going. The parents soon found that, by concentrating on the meaning of the textbooks and explaining terms and words their children found difficult, they were perfectly able to help their children. Similarly, when the children came to write up their assignments, the write-and-spell experience stood them in good stead. Not only were the parents a resource of help, advice and encouragement, the challenge of the unrealistic demands made upon some of the children was seen not as a deterrent but as a stimulus. Later many parents were able to report on the marked improvement there had been in their children's school work as a result.

A Sub-project in Schools

Although the Teacher-Researcher visited the parents at least once a fortnight it was soon apparent that ideally more frequent visits were needed by some parents with heavy family or employment commitments. Some parents, too, were less successful than others in helping their children with the activities. We decided to mount a sub-project in two schools to explore the possibility of how effectively the main design could be translated into schools and at the same time reduce the work-load of parents. Two schools for pupils aged 7–11 years agreed to take part. They were asked to identify pupils with severe reading difficulties in the 7-year-old age-group. The parents of these children were asked to carry out paired-reading; the teachers were asked to undertake the activities based on the reading. The sub-project successfully helped the children's reading in both schools. One school found that the children made such progress that parents and staff were keen to extend the sub-project for a further term and to involve more children and parents. This proved so successful and popular that the methods were extended to cover all pupils needing help in reading in the school.

Evaluation of the Project

What proved of greatest value was regressing the children to a level of reading at which they were secure. Using parents was also a considerable success. Some found it hard to sustain efforts for a whole year and some found it virtually impossible to do more than encourage. For the majority it was considered a rich and re-warding, if demanding, experience. The paired-reading and prepared reading approaches also made a major contribution. After the success of the intervention with the homework diffi-culties, guided reading, in which the parent first checked that the books were within the child's ability, was the natural development for some pupils.

Every one of the activities, such as write-and-spell, the coding, or the nonsense rhymes, was considered by some children to have helped them greatly or most of all. By the same token, of course, some children did not enjoy some of the activities and they were dropped as soon as this became apparent. Test results showed that all the children had made progress in spelling but, inevitably, for some this still lagged behind their progress in reading.

The Holiday Schools were remarkably successful so far as the children were concerned. The majority enjoyed being with other children with similar problems and they enjoyed working with the teachers. All but two said they would like to come to more Holiday Schools after the project was over. The two who said they would rather stay at home and play were children who, it had been found, had other difficulties in addition to their reading and learning problems. That they made the progress they did in the year was itself remarkable. Although the three holiday Schools provided only a maximum of 31 hours instruction in reading, as compared with the maximum of 180 hours instruction at home, many of the children and a few of the parents, thought the Schools helped them significantly.

None of the parents or children attributed any of the success in reading to the children's ordinary schools. Support is given to this view by the disappointing performance of the pupils in the Control Group. As the Dyslexic and Matched Groups of pupils enjoyed working with the teachers in the Holiday Schools it would appear that the methods employed in the ordinary schools are inappropriate to the needs of the children or that, if the methods are appropriate, the children are not being given enough individual attention. When a holistic approach was applied in the sub-project schools, and when parents and teachers worked in harmony with one another, however, everyone benefited and the pupils made significant and rapid progress.

Finally, whether or not the children were classified as dyslexic made no difference to the benefit they derived from the project. The parents of the dyslexic pupils saw the project as the first practical help they had received and, in the termly meetings they attended together with the parents of the Matched Group pupils, made it clear that their anxieties and concern for their children had diminished once they were given something to do which gave their children success in reading. All parents urged that there should be more such projects, that help and guidance should be given much earlier, that more support should be given than we had been able to provide to parents whose commitments were such that they had difficulty in keeping the programme going, and that the advice they would give to other parents was to persevere — the children can learn to read.

Realizing the Right to Read

Whatever the merits or demerits of the holistic approach to reading which we used with the parents of the dyslexic and severely reading retarded readers, what was interesting was that they found it easier to understand than we had anticipated. As one father commented; "It makes sense". Some of the remedial teacher-advisers, however, quite properly questioned our reliance on a holistic approach when all the research evidence and their own experience pointed to the importance of a structured and phonic method. It was only later that they realized that by learning to read by reading and by learning to write and spell by writing, the children were, in fact, becoming thoroughly familiar with all the strategies they considered so essential. It is a tribute to their professionalism that they co-operated from the start by suppressing their own inclinations and, at the end of the project, indicated that they could see its value and relevance to the needs of these and similar pupils. Like the teachers in the sub-project school which had found the approach so successful, they had nothing but praise and admiration for the contribution the parents had made.

We are quite convinced that, if more children are to make more progress in reading, if early difficulties are to be quickly and effectively overcome, and if more children are to be prevented from labouring for years with their difficulties in reading, writing and spelling, then it is essential that all parents who are able and willing should be encouraged to read to and with their children and to hear them read. Some parents will need little help or encouragement, others will need help and encouragement according to their changing or perennial difficulties. Some parents will find that helping their children improves their own reading and other skills, while others will need help from another member of the family or someone who can give a few minutes every day. Most parents can give encouragement and take an interest in their children's progress. One parent was so busy that her twelve-year-old daughter took over complete responsibility for her own programme and homework and made excellent progress; in another large family, the boy's prepared reading consisted of reading to his younger brothers and sisters when they were in bed. Of course there must be flexibility, and it would be senseless to suggest that all parents are the best natural educators of their own children. *All we are advocating is that rather than alienating parents or regarding them as passive partners they are welcomed as active contributors to their children's education and to helping their children to learn to read, write and spell.*

Reading subjects at University — and at School

If this is to be done, however, there must be much more flexibility and resourcefulness in schools. Too many parents have been patronized and patted on the head and told not to fuss or worry — or to come back in six months' time — for too long. The aura of mystique and of esoteric and recondite practices, which is as much the protective camouflage of the educational as of any other profession, is completely unjustified so far as the teaching of reading is concerned.

Schools need to remember, too, that it is no accident of language that students go to universities to *read* subjects. It is commonly assumed that children learn to read somewhere in their first years of schooling and that that is the end of the matter. Learning to read is a continuing process and every educator of children has the responsibility of fostering its development. Every subject teacher is not a teacher of English, save in the most general sense, but every subject teacher has a responsbility to develop the reading and language skills particular to that subject. Expecting children to read textbooks which are manifestly beyond their capabilities is simply failing to teach the subject to the children. If standards of literacy are to rise and the educational needs of children are to be met, then subjects teachers should either dispense with the difficult textbooks and provide books and assignments within the capabilities of the children, or contribute what they can to helping the children to master the skills they demand of them. If they have the humility to accept that this will stretch their own capabilities and resources then they should seek the resources of the goodwill and human energy of the parents and their colleagues. But consigning children to remedial classes and units without first delineating the specific vocabularies or concepts in which the pupils need help assumes that others can take over their responsibilities.

Teachers are not employed to occupy the children but to teach them. The only measure of their effectiveness is in what the children learn from them. If the children fail to learn the values, skills, concepts, facts and ways of thinking appropriate to an area of knowledge they have not been taught appropriately. Central to all knowledge is language. No one who teaches can escape the responsibility of developing the language and language skills of the children they teach. Reading subjects in schools, therefore, has to be seen in a new perspective if the needs of the children with whom we are concerned are to be met and if standards of literacy are to be raised. There is a shortage of books in most subject areas which are appropriate to the needs of these and many other pupils for a

controlled vocabulary and syntax. There is, too, an absence of
expertise in developing the abilities of 20 per cent of the school
population across the curriculum above the level of basic functional
literacy.

While this remain the case we will continue to produce future
generations of parents whose skills of reading, writing and spelling
are so inadequate and insecure that they will be unable either to
contribute fully to our complex technological society or to the early
education of their own children. Genetics will not be to blame for
that.

Children as Active Partners

The children who were helped to read by the project enjoyed the
Holiday Schools, showed a remarkable capacity for work and
enjoyed working with their teachers. For a long time many of them
had been unhappy in their own schools and certainly working far
below their levels of ability. Failure in reading had reduced them to
a state of "work paralysis"; success in reading had transformed
them to a state, to use another of Erik Erikson's apt terms, "of active
apprenticeship". They began to make quite rapid progress in their
ordinary schools, in many cases, as a result. In the majority of these
cases this in turn was commented upon favourably by their
teachers. Not all pupils were fortunate. One child struggled to write
a verse for homework only to have it torn up by the teacher with the
words: "I'm not wasting my time trying to read that!" But, while
that was untypical of what happens when children are trying and
in part succeeding, it illustrates the kind of attitude which made
many of the children unhappy *when* they were failing. As many
parents in both groups commented, what had hurt and offended
them was not merely that their children were regarded as stupid by
their peers and as failures by their teachers, attitudes they could
understand, but that nobody cared, nobody took any interest.

These children, of course, are not alone in this respect. Although
the majority of schools are caring communities, there are others in
which the "hidden curriculum" of the school makes it clear to the
pupils that they are failures only fit for the worst teachers, the worst
form-rooms, the most watered-down curriculum, the narrowest
range of subjects. Or they are fully integrated and almost totally

ignored. What we learned from working with these children was there was another resource of energy and goodwill still largely untapped. It was the children themselves. Fifteen dyslexic and fifteen reading retarded boys and girls, all strangers to one another and to their teachers, from as diverse social backgrounds as one could meet in any large school, aged between 8 and 13 years, walked into a strange school and settled down to work in the middle of their holidays. Why?

The reason was that they had been transformed, by their parents' work with them, from failures to successful and self-improving readers and were now motivated to learn and to achieve. They were now active participants in learning, eager to master reading. They had learned that the only true motivation for learning is the need to learn. They had been helped by their parents to learn more than how to read: they had learned to learn and to accept responsibility for their own survival and for their own futures.

Dyslexia and Learning

The concept of dyslexia as a specific learning difficulty in reading is a useful but misleading one. Its utility, quite apart from whatever legal and administrative purposes it may serve, lies in the fact that it states clearly in everyday language the apparent problems of the children. It is misleading in that it suggests the difficulties are specific to reading, writing and spelling. The difficulties are, however, in the vast majority of cases, in learning itself. As we have seen, many children with all the "soft" signs and characteristics of dyslexic children, are successful readers. Dyslexic pupils are taught to read despite their cross-modal integration, glue-ears, auditory and visual sequential memory and other problems. What distinguishes dyslexic and severely reading retarded children from children with similar constitutional or environmental difficulties who can read, is that they have failed to learn efficient strategies to overcome or circumvent their difficulties and have stopped trying to learn. Initial difficulties and initial failure have led to confusion which is compounded by retreat from reading and withdrawal from the participant act of active learning. The children learn to be failures in reading, persist in using only their inefficient strategies and, not surprisingly, their difficulties are said to be intractable. Having cut a path through the jungle of their difficulties which has led them to an unscalable mountain, they stick to their path.

If we accept that their difficulties are real enough, although possibly avoidable had they been detected or handled differently at the time, we will not address ourselves to the difficulties but to the children and their learning in that order. Frequently we have advised teachers of children with a variety of physical, intellectual and emotional difficulties, to stop teaching them and, instead, to stand back and try to see the world from the children's standpoint. We have suggested that from their knowledge of the children and their situations, they ask themselves how they would feel, think and respond, and what would stimulate and motivate them. Then, we have suggested that they ask the children what they are really interested in, what they really want to learn. The next step is to prove to them that we can teach them to get what they want. Instead of finding out what they can't do and giving them a hell of a lot of it, we need to find what they can do or want to do and give them the sense of achievement in doing it. If we can't teach them to read, then let us teach them to swim or play dominoes or whatever. But whatever we do, we need to show them that we can teach and that they can learn. In doing this we will, at least, divert them from plodding on down their path through the jungle. If none of this is possible, we can certainly stop trying to teach them what they cannot do and we can start building up their self-confidence and respect in activities in which they are reasonably competent. The child who has bruised knees and hands from falling off his bike doesn't want to be stuck back on it straight away, but needs time for the scars and bruises to heal. Nor does he want a lesson about the sprockets, chains and ball-bearings or the physics of locomotion.

The next step is to take the children right off their old paths and to give them success in learning new ones to achievement in reading. We must take them right back to where they are really secure and show them how successful they can be at that level. Some will need a lot of real achievement at that level, others only a little. From then on, we should make sure that the approach we are using leads them well away from their old paths and continuously builds success upon success. Only in this way will they become active and self-motivated learners. During this process we may well reward their successes with certificates of achievement or posters of their pop-stars, but we will be, above all, nurturing their own intrinsic feelings of learning to learn again and being motivated by the need to achieve and to master. Fortunately, as we have seen, there are many paths to reading whether by language experience or look-and-say, but all paths must converge upon meaning. Once we have shown children that that is where they are going they will become self-improving and reading will become self-rewarding.

If we conceptualize children's difficulties as learning difficulties, then we owe it to them to show them how to learn. The danger of regarding dyslexia as a specific learning difficulty in reading which is cognitive in essence, genetically determined and representing a specific maturational defect, however, it may be defined to reflect current fashions, is that *we won't see the children for the jargon*. With so many preconceptions about what may or may not be their difficulties we are in danger of seeing only their deficits and none of their abilities. We project upon these children our own uncertainties, the inadequacy of our own understanding, and conceal them beneath a veil of vague verbiage. It is even more dangerous if, in search of precision and clarity, we go on to exclude intellectual, emotional or socio-cultural factors. If children have a cognitive difficulty and a maturational lag then, if these words mean anything, they must have intellectual difficulties. If they have known years of failure, emotional factors must be involved. If their schooling has failed to identify their needs and to meet them because they were ignored or ill-served by teachers whose understanding of the process of reading was inadequate, then socio-cultural factors are involved.

What understanding we do have of genetics does not support the Lamarckian view that acquired skills and characteristics are inherited. Genetics does tell us that each individual is unique. We must accept and welcome the fact that each child is different and that different children learn at different rates and in different ways. As parents and as educators we must provide for this diversity. We must also recognize that genetics tells us that each child is programmed to survive. As parents and as educators we must nourish and foster that drive to survive and to succeed in our complex literate society. What is curious about man is his curiosity. If some of our children have difficulties in learning to read we must give them the confidence and self-esteem to be curious and questing, to be motivated to learn by learning and to learn to read by reading.

Conclusion: What Must Be Done

The proper anxiety of parents, the curiosity of researchers and the concern of society for the literacy of our children have focused attention upon the need for a more dynamic model of the process of reading and for a deeper understanding of learning. We have attempted to show how a holistic model of reading in which writing and spelling go hand in hand is as appropriate to culturally deprived, emotionally disturbed, intellectually impaired, severely reading retarded or physically handicapped children as it is to dyslexic children. Our view is that all children are special and have special needs and that only an adequate theory of reading, allied to adequate theories of development and instruction will serve all their needs.

There is much that we still do not know about the difficulties some children experience and much that we need to know before our theories are adequate. But we know enough to do more than we are doing. If we recognize all children's right to read then we must raise standards of literacy above the merely functional level for millions of pupils and adults so that they can benefit from and contribute what they can to society and to the education of their own children. We must use the resources of educational plant that lies empty and idle for a fifth of the year. We must equip teachers with a more rigorous and efficient repertoire of skills, techniques and resources, and a deeper understanding of the children they teach and of reading. We must harness the natural concern and understanding of parents, whenever they are able to do so, to initiate and to foster the development of their children's reading. We must give help and guidance to those parents who, for whatever reason, need it so that their children are in no way disadvantaged. We must welcome the children who have particular needs in our schools, identify those needs early, and effectively meet them. And we must harness the need to learn and to achieve in all our children as partners in the process of cultural transmission, development and change. In the process of the mediation and facilitation of children's learning, which is education, *we* have a unique opportunity to learn. Our children are society's greatest resource of human energy and goodwill. We must give them all, not labels, but the right to read.

Appendix

Playing the Language Game — A Holistic Model of Reading
Development

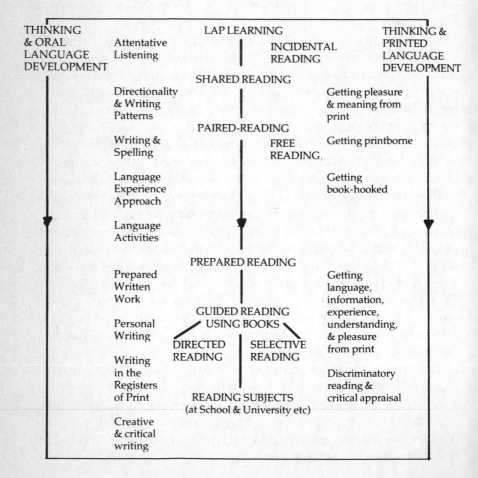

The language of the child contributes to and is developed by reading.
Starting from listening to and then following the adult, reading for
meaning develops hand in hand with the patterns of writing and of
spelling. "Language experience" approaches develop these encoding
skills as the print-borne child develops the decoding skills and cues to
meaning. Writing and language games and activities based on the
reading ensure reinforcement of these skills. Throughout, the emphasis
is on meaning, on learning to learn and on the motivation of learning by
the child's need to find out, to achieve and to master. The interaction of
the adult ensures success at all times and keeps the rate of progress in
harmony with those needs and with the developing skills of the child.

Lap learning: Rhymes, jingles, songs and listening to parent read
                   in the security of lap or knee.
Incidental reading: Names, street signs, posters; environmental print.
Shared reading: Child listens to parent read and follows finger on
                   page and from page to page. Child interacts with
                   questions and answers.
Paired-reading: Parent talks about passage, reads aloud passage;
                   parent and child read in unison; they read the same
                   passage with pauses for child to supply next word/s;
                   child reads same passage aloud alone but is helped
                   as necessary.
Prepared reading: Parent talks about and reads passage aloud with
                   child following. Child then reads same passage
                   silently and asks for any words not known or under-
                   stood. Child reads same passage aloud alone but
                   helped as necessary. This is a transition to in-
                   dependent reading; in the later stages the child is
                   only asked to read aloud texts within his capability or
                   texts he has read silently and been given words or
                   meanings about which there is uncertainty.
Guided reading: The child is given books, from, say, a series or,
                   preferably, selected according to interests and
                   ability, which progressively extend and develop
                   reading skill.
Using books: Using newspapers, magazines, dictionaries, atlases,
                   directories, information books, etc., to find out.
Directed reading: After oral preparation of subject matter child is given
                   passage or chapter to read. The beginning and
                   development of use of books for study which
                   continues throughout the education process. New
                   skills are developed here, such as skipping,
                   skimming, identifying argument, reasoning, etc.

Free reading: Vital voracious stage when everything is read from
                        comics to novels; reading in bed or curled up in a
                        corner. Stage at which parents once told children
                        they would wear eyes out.

Reading subjects   Directed reading for which each subject teacher or
across the   lecturer is responsible for the development of pupil's
curriculum: ability to use appropriate skills, values, concepts,
                        etc of the body of knowledge concerned, e.g., read-
                        ing chemistry textbooks requires different skills
                        from reading Chaucer.

   The stages of progression should not be seen as hierarchical or as one
stage strictly following in dependent order upon the previous stage.
"Reading subjects" may well begin in the "Shared reading" stage if the
child is listening to a book about dinosaurs or dragon-flies; "Free
reading" frequently begins before the child is print-borne. Rather, the
stages represent a basic and essential developmental progressions towards mastery for pupils who have difficulty in learning to read. Able
readers may start with "Free reading" and their spelling may never catch
up! The hyperlexic, perhaps?
   The holistic model is essentially preventative of difficulties arising.
When applied to children or adults who have already experienced years
of failure and difficulty they should be taken back to the stage at which
they are completely secure and able to be successful. It is then essential to
adapt the activities of that stage so that they are appropriate to their
maturity and interests. Thus, illiterate adults only secure at the "lap
learning" stage might well begin with conversation about the advertise-
ments, jingles, road signs etc. with which they are thoroughly familiar at
the recognition level.

Glossary

acquired dyslexia:
loss or impairment of the ability to read as the result of damage to the brain.

alexia:
now used as synonymous with acquired dyslexia.

aphasia:
loss or impairment of the ability to use speech or understand language; *expressive aphasia:* difficulties in using language in speech; *receptive aphasia:* difficulties in understanding speech; *global aphasia:* difficulties in using and understanding all forms of language; also "dysphasia".

basal readers:
in North America, series of graded primers.

blending:
sounding letters together, e.g. *br-, -ft, ba-, -ed.*

cerebral dominance:
the establishment in one side or hemisphere of the brain of the main areas involved in language; usually the left hemisphere is dominant.

cross-modal integration:
the efficient transfer of perceived information from one sense or modality to others, e.g., relating what is heard with what is seen or vice versa.

cross-laterality:
using the eye, ear or foot on the opposite side of the body from the preferred hand, e.g. left-handed but using right eye or ear or foot. Hence *mixed-laterality* when, say, the preferred use is right hand, left eye, right ear and left foot.

deep dyslexia: reading difficulties in phonemic decoding observed in cases of alexia; patients make meaningful substitutions for difficult words, suggesting that the right hemisphere, which is undamaged, is interceding.

deep structure of language: the meaning of language, not its sound, print or grammar; the deep structure of two sentences may be the same but their *surface structures* may differ, e.g. "The dog chased the car" and "The car was chased by the dog".

diacritics: marks attached to letters to indicate pronunciation, e.g. café; used in teaching of reading to distinguish the sounds of letters, e.g. mát, māte.

digraphs: two letters making one sound; a two-letter phoneme; consonantal digraphs such as *th, ch, ph,* and vowel digraphs such as *ea, ou, oo.*

dyscalculia: also acalculia; difficulties in arithmetical calculations.

dysgraphia: difficulties in handwriting; also agraphia.

dyslexia: difficulties in reading and spelling; short for *specific developmental dyslexia* when applied to children, when it suggests a constitutional causation but with no implication of brain damage in contradistinction to acquired dyslexia or alexia.

EEG: electroencephalogram: the recording of variations in the electrical potential of the brain from electrodes attached to the scalp.

functional literacy: the minimal level of efficiency in reading and writing necessary for effective participation in and contribution to a society.

grapheme: minimal written or printed units of language; a letter or combination of letters representing a phoneme; e.g. *A, a* and *a* are three graphemes, as are *qu-, kn-* and *pn-.*

holistic approach to reading: concerned with the whole or totality of the reading process and indicating that the process is both more than the sum of its parts and that it should be taught as a language activity in which meaning is decoded from print and encoded in writing and spelling.

linguistics: the scientific study of language.

morpheme: the minimal units of meaning in a language; a word or part of a word which has meaning, e.g. *book/s, book/ed, book/ing, bi-, dis-, dys-, -ly, -ness* are all morphemes.

phoneme: the minimal sound unit of a language, e.g. *o* is a phoneme represented by a number of graphemes such as *toe* and *boat*.

phonetics: the scientific study of the sounds of language.

phonics: teaching reading by emphasizing the importance of the sounds of letters, their blends and combinations, to build up words.

primer reading age: assessment of children's reading ability according to the level of difficulty of the primers they are reading efficiently.

primers: series of graded first reading books.

psycholinguistics: psychological aspects of language; the study of linguistic behaviour in relation to acquiring language, attention, memory, perception, etc.

reading age (RA): assessment of children's reading ability as measured by a standardized reading test, e.g., RA 10 yrs means that a child has scored at the level of the average 10-year-olds on the same test; of very limited value, misleading and based on misconceptions of reading process, child development and psychological measurement.

rebus: originally a punning puzzle in which a word is represented by pictures, e.g. a cat on a log for catalogue; adapted for use in teaching reading by pictograms and signs as in the Peabody Rebus Reading Programme.

retardation in reading: whereas "backwardness in reading" means that a child is reading at a level below that of other children of the same age, retardation means that a child is reading at a level below that of children of the same age *and of the same level of ability*, e.g., a child aged 10 yrs and IQ 120 is expected to read at the 12-year-old level $(10 \times 120 \div 100 = 12 \text{ yrs})$ and if he, in fact, only reads at the 9-year-old level (RA 9 yrs) then he is 3 yrs $(12 - 9 \text{ yrs})$ retarded in reading; many psychologists manage without this notion and its underlying assumptions, preferring to focus attention upon the children's need to read, whatever the level of their so-called abilities or intelligence.

reversals: reversing letters, *b* for *d*, *q*, for *p*, or words *on* for *no*, *dog* for *god*; mirror writing; a common phenomenon in under 7s, and some under 9s, and in adults under stress.

saccadic eye-movements: grass-hopper-like leaps backwards and forwards of the eyes when scanning a picture or reading a line of print.

specific reading retardation: (see "reading retardation" above), used to distinguish pupils whose reading difficulties cannot be accounted for by lack of general ability ("intelligence") or opportunity or other factors such as visual or hearing difficulties; favoured by some psychologists and educationalists in preference to "specific developmental dyslexia" with which it is synonymous in use; when degree of retardation is "measured", multiple-regression equations are used to allow for the differing characteristics of the tests used to "measure" reading and ability.

strephosymbolia: the "twisting of symbols"; mirror writing or reversals; thought by Orton to be a charactersitic of word-blind children.

surface structure of language: the sound, visual and grammatical representation and characteristics of language in contradistinction to its *deep structure* (c.v.) or meaning.

syndrome: a characteristic pattern or group of symptoms.

syntax: a branch of grammar concerned with sentence structure and the rules governing the relationship between words in a sentence.

word-blindness: from the German "wortblindheit" and synonymous with dyslexia; "congenital word-blindness", like "developmental dyslexia", being applied to children.

References & Further Reading

ASHTON-WARNER, S. (1963) *Teacher*. London: Secker & Warburg.
BRUNER, J.S. (1966) *Toward a Theory of Instruction*. Cambridge, Mass: Harvard University Press.
BRUNER, J.S. (1971) *The Relevance of Education*. London: Geo. Allen & Unwin.
BRUNER, J.S. (1973) *Beyond the Information Given*. London: Geo. Allen & Unwin.
CENTRAL ADVISORY COUNCIL FOR EDUCATION (1967) *Children and their Primary Schools*, (The Plowden Report), London: HMSO.
CHAPMAN, J.L., HOFFMAN, M. and MERRITT, J.E. (1974) *Developing Fluent Reading*. Milton Keynes: Open University Press.
CIPOLLA, C.M. (1969) *Literacy & Development in the West*. London: Penguin.
CLAY, M.M. (1979) *The Early Detection of Reading Difficulties*. Auckland: Heinemann Educational Books.
COLTHEART, M., PATTERSON, K. and MARSHALL, J.C. (1980) *Deep Dyslexia*. London: Routledge & Kegan Paul.
CRYSTAL, D., FLETCHER, P. and GARMAN, M. (1976) *The Grammatical Analysis of Language Disability*. London: Edward Arnold.
CRYSTAL, D. (1979) *Working with LARSP*. London: Edward Arnold.
DALGLISH, C. (1982) *Illiteracy & the Offender*. Cambridge: Huntingdon Publications.
DANIELS, J.C. and DIACK, H. (1958) *The Standard Reading Tests*. London: Chatto and Windus.
DEPARTMENT OF EDUCATION AND SCIENCE (1972) *Children with Specific Reading Difficulties*. (The Tizard Report). London: HMSO.
DEPARTMENT OF EDUCATION AND SCIENCE (1975) *A Language for Life*. (The Bullock Report). London: HMSO.
DEPARTMENT OF EDUCATION AND SCIENCE (1978) *Special Educational Needs* (The Warnock Report). London: HMSO.

DOWNING, J. (1972) "The cognitive clarity theory of learning". In: SOUTHGATE, V. (Ed.) *Literacy at all Levels*. London: Ward Lock Educational.

EDWARDS, P. (1978) *Reading Problems: Identification & Treatment*. London: Heinemann Educational Books.

ERIKSON, E.H. (1965) *Childhood and Society*. London: Penguin.

ERIKSON, E.H. (1971) *Identity, Youth & Crisis*. London: Faber & Faber.

FERNALD, G. (1943) *Remedial Techniques in Basic School Subjects*. New York: McGraw-Hill.

FEUERSTEIN, R. (1980) *Instrumental Enrichment*. Baltimore: University Park Press.

GOODMAN, K.S. (1967) "Reading: A psycholinguistic guessing game". In: SINGER, H. and RUDDELL, R.B. (Eds), (1970) *Theoretical Models of Reading*. Delaware: International Reading Association.

GOODMAN, K.S. (1973) "Psycholinguistic universals in the reading process". In: SMITH, F. (1973) *Psycholinguistics and Reading*. London: Holt, Rinehart & Winston.

KIRK, S.A., McCARTHY, J.J. and KIRK, W.D. (1971) *Illinois Test of Psycholinguistic Abilities*. Urbana: University of Illinois Press.

LAWTON, D. (1981) *An Introduction to Teaching and Learning*. London: Hodder & Stoughton.

LUNZER, E.A. and MORRIS, J.F. (1968) *Development in Human Learning*. London: Staples Press.

LURIA, A.R. (1973) *The Working Brain: An Introduction to Neuropsychology*. London: Penguin.

MILES, T.R. (1978) *Understanding Dyslexia*. London: Hodder & Stoughton, Teach Yourself Books.

NEALE, M.D. (1966) *The Neale Analysis of Reading Ability*. London: Macmillan.

NEWTON, M.J., THOMSPON, M.E. and RICHARDS, I.L. (1979) *Readings in Dyslexia: A study text to accompany The Aston Index*. Wisbech: Learning Development Aids.

PAVLIDIS, G.T. and MILES, T.R. (Ed.), (1981) *Dyslexia Research and its Application to Education*. Chichester: John Wiley & Sons.

RAVENETTE, A.T. (1968) *Dimensions of Reading Difficulties*. Oxford: Pergamon Press.

RUTTER, M., TIZARD, S. and WHITMORE, K. (1970) *Education, Health and Behaviour*. London: Longman.

RUTTER, M. and YULE, W. (1973) "Specific Reading Retardation", in MANN, L. and SABATINO, D. (Eds) *The First Review of Special Education*. USA: Battonwood Farms.

SMITH, F. (1971) *Understanding Reading: A Psycholinguistic Analysis of Reading and Learning to Read*. London: Holt, Reinhart & Winston.

SMITH, F. (1973) *Psycholinguistics and Reading*. London: Holt, Reinhart & Winston.

SMITH, F. (1978) *Reading*. Cambridge: Cambridge University Press.

SOUTHGATE, V., ARMOLD, H. and JOHNSON, S. (1981) *Extending Beginning Reading*. London: Heinemann Educational Books.

STAUFFER, R. (1970) *The Language Experience Approach to The Teaching of Reading*. New York: Harper Row.

STOTT, D.H. (1978) *Helping Children with Learning Difficulties*. London: Ward Lock Educational.

STRANG, R. (1968) "Research to improve the teaching of reading.". In: MORRIS, J. (1968) *The First R*. London: Ward Lock Educational.

STRANG, R. (1969) *Diagnostic Teaching of Reading*. New York: McGraw-Hill.

TANSLEY, P. and PANCKHURST, J. (1981) *Children with Specific Learning Difficulties*. Windsor: NFER-Nelson Publishing Co.

VELLUTINO, F.R. (1979) *Dyslexia, Theory and Research*. Cambridge, Mass: The MIT Press.

VERNON, M.D. (1957) *Backwardness in Reading*. Cambridge: Cambridge University Press.

VERNON, M.D. (1971) *Reading and its Difficulties*. Cambridge: Cambridge University Press.

VYGOTSKY, L.S. (Tr. 1962) *Thought and Language*. Cambridge, Mass: The MIT Press.

WEBER, K.J. (1978) *Yes, They Can!* Milton Keynes: Open University Press.

WEBER, K.J. (1982) *The Teacher is the Key: A practical guide for teaching adolescents with learning difficulties*. Milton Keynes: Open University Press.

YOUNG, P. (1970) *Data on Reading*. Huddersfield, Schofield & Sims.

YOUNG, P. and J. (1978) *Write and Spell*. Edinburgh: Oliver & Boyd.

YOUNG, P. and TYRE, C. (1985) *Teach Your Child to Read: The Good Parents' Guide to Reading, Writing and Spelling*. London: Fontana Paperbacks.

Index

Numbers in bold type refer to entries in *'References and Further Reading'*.

173